Economic evaluation of interventions for occupational health and safety

Economic evaluation of interventions for occupational health and safety
Developing good practice

Edited by

Emile Tompa
Scientist,
Institute for Work & Health,
Toronto, Canada

Anthony J. Culyer
Chair of Health Policy and System Design
University of Toronto, Canada
and
Professor of Economics,
University of York, United Kingdom

Roman Dolinschi
Economist,
Institute for Work & Health,
Toronto, Canada

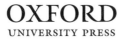

OXFORD
UNIVERSITY PRESS

OXFORD

UNIVERSITY PRESS

Great Clarendon Street, Oxford OX2 6DP

Oxford University Press is a department of the University of Oxford.
It furthers the University's objective of excellence in research, scholarship,
and education by publishing worldwide in

Oxford New York

Auckland Cape Town Dar es Salaam Hong Kong Karachi
Kuala Lumpur Madrid Melbourne Mexico City Nairobi
New Delhi Shanghai Taipei Toronto

With offices in

Argentina Austria Brazil Chile Czech Republic France Greece
Guatemala Hungary Italy Japan Poland Portugal Singapore
South Korea Switzerland Thailand Turkey Ukraine Vietnam

Oxford is a registered trade mark of Oxford University Press
in the UK and in certain other countries

Published in the United States
by Oxford University Press Inc., New York

British Library Cataloguing in Publication Data

Data available

Library of Congress Cataloguing in Publication Data

Data available

Typeset by Cepha Imaging Private Ltd., Bangalore, India
Printed in Great Britain
on acid-free paper by
Biddles Ltd., King's Lynn, Norfolk

ISBN 978-0-19-953359-6

10 9 8 7 6 5 4 3 2 1

Whilst every effort has been made to ensure that the contents of this book are as complete,
accurate and up-to-date as possible at the date of writing, Oxford University Press is not able
to give any guarantee or assurance that such is the case. Readers are urged to take appropriately
qualified medical advice in all cases. The information in this book is intended to be useful to
the general reader, but should not be used as a means of self-diagnosis or for the prescription
of mediciation. The opinions expressed throughout the book are those of the contributors,
and not the organizations they work for.

Preface

In assessments of the research literature on the economic evaluation of occupational health and safety (OHS) interventions, one increasingly meets phrases such as: 'understanding of economic techniques ... was limited', 'significant methodological limitations', 'a complete absence of cost-effectiveness or cost–benefit analysis', 'lack of competency within the health and safety professions in techniques of economic evaluation', and 'well-designed and conducted evaluations of program costs and benefits were nearly impossible to find' (all quotes come from Niven 2002). Other reviews of the OHS literature, including our own, have arrived at similar conclusions (DeRango and Franzini 2003; Goossens *et al.* 1999; Tompa *et al.* 2007c).

Undertaking economic evaluations of OHS interventions can be difficult for a number of reasons:

- the policy arena of OHS and labour legislation is complex, with multiple stakeholders and sometimes conflicting incentives and priorities;

- there are substantial differences in the perceptions of health risks associated with work experiences amongst workplace parties, policymakers and other OHS stakeholders;

- there is consequential lack of consensus about what, in principle, ought to count as a benefit or cost of intervening or not intervening;

- the burden of costs and consequences may be borne by various stakeholders in the system;

- there are multiple providers of indemnity and medical care coverage, such that no one measure accurately captures the full cost of work-related injury and illness, nor conversely, the benefits of their prevention;

- industry-specific human resources practices (e.g., hiring temporary workers and self-employed contractors, farming out non-core activities) can make it difficult to identify all work-related injuries and illnesses;

- in general, there is an absence of good guidelines regarding costs and consequences combined with a dearth of data available from organizations making it both challenging and expensive to obtain good measures.

The above list of reasons might explain why few studies of OHS interventions contain an economic evaluation and why the quality of economic evaluations in the few that do attempt it is usually poor.

Hindering the advancement of the application of economic evaluation methods in OHS is the fact there is very little focused methods guidance available to OHS researchers. Most methods books are designed for use in a clinical setting which is a very different context. A recent conference co-organized by the National Institute for Occupational Safety and Health (NIOSH) and the World Health Organization (WHO) gathered members of the global OHS community to discuss methods and practice in the economic evaluation of health and safety interventions and programmes at the company level (Eijkemans and Fingerhut 2005). The call for this type of meeting underlines the importance of the topic, yet although the conference proceedings were published in a special issue of the *Journal of Safety Research*, no economic evaluation methods text has yet been designed expressly for use in evaluating OHS interventions. This book has been developed to fill this gap. It is designed to lay the foundations for a systematic methodology of economic evaluation of OHS interventions, to identify the main barriers to research of high quality and practical relevance, and to propose a research strategy to remedy these weaknesses.

The book is meant to serve researchers, practitioners, policymakers, and course instructors who are familiar with the nature of initiatives undertaken to improve OHS performance, and the evaluation of the effectiveness of such initiatives. In general, individuals interested in undertaking, commissioning, teaching, learning about, or appraising economic evaluations of OHS interventions will find something of interest in this book. We have assumed that readers may come from various fields, including OHS practitioners, ergonomists, engineers, occupational health clinicians, health promotion consultants, workplace studies researchers, applied economists, and instructors of economic evaluation methods and topics in OHS studies. We have tried to write the book accordingly.

We have also attempted to make the book broadly applicable in jurisdictions having different institutional and regulatory approaches to OHS, disability policy, and health care provision. One chapter in the book is a survey of the institutional and regulatory context in several jurisdictions, included to provide readers with a sense of how widely the context can vary, and how different systems can affect workplace parties and other stakeholders in different ways.

Our book requires some familiarity with issues related to economic evaluation, although it is not meant to serve only a specialist audience (i.e., economists). Although the book is intended to prepare readers for hands-on experiences in undertaking economic evaluations of OHS interventions, it is not intended to be a methodological 'cookbook', through which the novice can learn to undertake an economic evaluation. It is a supplement to, rather than a replacement of, introductory texts to economic evaluation such as Drummond *et al.* (2005). Our main focus has been on those OHS matters where the application of methods is different from its application in health care. For standard economic evaluation procedures, we provide up-to-date references.

The book is probably best read in conjunction with health technology methods texts such as Gold *et al.* (1996) and Drummond *et al.* (2005), and assessment of public health policies texts, such as Haddix *et al.* (2002). There is a thematic relationship with the text by Oxenburgh *et al.* (2004). However, that text differs from this in that it focuses on making the 'business case' for ergonomic interventions, whereas here we present a systematic methodology for economic evaluation of OHS interventions, accounting for multiple stakeholders and perspectives as well as the complexity of OHS policy. We include, but go beyond the production of 'business cases' for the consumption of firms. We have sought to extend economic evaluations of OHS interventions to higher levels, for example, ones that take account of the multiplicity of stakeholders, the diversity of issues that come to bear in the OHS policy arena, and the more ultimate consideration of general social welfare.

There are three clusters of topics in the book—scene setting and context chapters; specific topic chapters; and a concluding chapter with suggestions for a 'reference case'. The scene setting and context chapters provide a wealth of background material ranging from a presentation of the broad conceptualization of work and health to suggestions for strategies in confronting the data dearth often experienced by OHS researchers. Lessons are also drawn from other literatures, primarily the health technology assessment literature and that on valuing reductions in physical risk. A discussion of the value of health and safety, and a critical review of the OHS literature provide a platform for developing insight and guidance on how to take the application of economic evaluation methods further in future studies.

The specific topic chapters delve into the principles and application of economic evaluation methods with focus on issues most salient to OHS. Study design, type of analysis, costs, consequences, uncertainty and equity feature in the roster of topics that provide guidance on analytical and decision-making challenges.

In the final chapter we synthesize the summaries, conclusions, challenges, and recommendations from across the book. Drawing primarily from the list of recommendations provided at the end of each specific topic chapter, we develop and present a 'reference case.' This is intended to serve as a minimal set of criteria for which we judge there to be a professional scientific consensus. One benefit of standardization, beyond encouraging good practice, is that it makes results from different studies more readily comparable in future evaluations. We think it is worth trying to build such a professional scientific consensus based on a reasoned attempt to distil what government, workers, workers' families, employers, workers' compensation boards, health and safety regulators, and other third party payers, indeed, all stakeholders, are seeking to achieve or—where there is disagreement—to identify more precisely what the disagreement may be about, and to assess its size and significance. Our prescriptions for a reference case serve as a starting point. As the application of economic evaluation in the OHS arena matures, the reference case may evolve as the distilling becomes more refined.

Emile Tompa
Anthony J. Culyer
Roman Dolinschi
2008

Acknowledgements

This book has been made possible by substantial contributions of time and effort from many individuals, and generous funding support from several organizations.

The initiative began in 2005 with a working group consisting of Tony Culyer, Roman Dolinschi, Jacob Etches, William Gnam, Michel Grignon, Audrey Laporte, and Emile Tompa. The working group met regularly for a period of approximately one year to develop the idea, identify a list potential contributing authors, and plan an international workshop to serve as a forum for peer review of contributions. The workshop, which was entitled 'Developing Good Practice in the Economic Evaluation of Workplace Interventions for Health and Safety,' was held in Toronto, Canada on April 6 and 7, 2006.

A number of people based at the Institute for Work & Health, Toronto, Canada, came together to secure funding for, plan and organize the international workshop, namely Jane Gibson, Lyudmila Mansurova, Cameron Mustard, Greer Palloo and Sandra Sinclair. Also supporting various activities at the workshop were Sudipa Bhattacharyya, Claire de Oliveira, Roman Dolinschi, Jacob Etches, Catherine Morris, and Anna Sarnocinska-Hart. We are very grateful for the time and effort of all involved in executing the workshop and ensuring that the two intense days of reviewing, critiquing and discussing were a success.

Funding for the international workshop was provided by the Institute for Work & Health (which receives core funding from the Workplace Safety and Insurance Board of Ontario), the German Hauptverband der gewerblichen Berufsgenossenschaften (HVBG), the umbrella organization that provides statutory accident insurance and prevention services to the private sector, and the Foundation for Research and Education in Work and Health Studies (an educational endowment fund created by the Institute for Work & Health). We thank these funders for their generous support of this initiative.

A number of academics contributed their time and expertise toward preparing material for this book. Their contributions are what made this book possible and were given pro bono to the initiative. The list of contributors is as follows: Ben Amick, Philip Bigelow, Alan Clayton, Donald Cole, Richard Cookson, Tony Culyer, Claire de Oliveira, Carolyn Dewa, Roman Dolinschi,

Peter Dorman, Dorte Eltard, William Gnam, Michel Grignon, Jeffrey Hoch, Ulrike Hotopp, Birgit Koeper, Thomas Kohstall, Audrey Laporte, John Mendeloff, Cameron Mustard, Karen Niven, Lynda Robson, Mark Sculpher, Sandra Sinclair, and Emile Tompa.

Several academics served as discussants at the workshop, again providing their time pro bono to the initiative, and we are very grateful for their critiques of the chapters. The discussants were Ben Amick, Donald Cole, Richard Cookson, Lori Curtis, Carolyn Dewa, Livio di Matteo, Peter Dorman, Kaj Frick, Jeffrey Hoch, Mark Sculpher, Jennifer Stewart, and Jean-Eric Tarride. Helpful comments for Chapter 5 were also provided by Michael Jones-Lee.

We are also indebted for the insightful commentary provided by seven anonymous reviewers, engaged by Oxford University Press. Their feedback has made the final product much stronger.

Finally, we thank Sara Morassaei who served as our editorial assistant and helped with preparation of the final manuscripts.

We extend our sincerest thanks to all involved in this initiative. The production of this book was truly a team effort.

Emile Tompa
Anthony J. Culyer
Roman Dolinschi

Contents

Part 3 **Conclusions**

Abbreviations

ASCC	Australian Safety and Compensation Council
CBA	cost–benefit analysis
CCA	cost–consequence analysis
CEA	cost-effectiveness analysis
CEAC	cost-effectiveness acceptability curve
CMA	cost-minimization analysis
CPP	Canada Pension Plan
CTD	cumulative trauma disorder
CUA	cost–utility analysis
CV	contingent valuation
DALY	Disability-Adjusted Life-Year
EU	European Union
FTE	full time equivalent
HRQL	health-related quality of life
HSC	Health and Safety Commission, United Kingdom
HSE	Health and Safety Executive, United Kingdom
HTA	health technology assessment
HYE	Healthy Year Equivalent
ICER	incremental cost-effectiveness ratio
INB	incremental net benefit
NHS	National Health Service, United Kingdom
NICE	National Institute for Health and Clinical Excellence, England and Wales
NIOSH	National Institute for Occupational Safety and Health, United States
NPV	net present value
OECD	Organization for Economic Cooperation and Development
OHS	occupational health and safety
OSHA	Occupational Safety and Health Administration, United States
PSA	probabilistic sensitivity analysis
QALY	Quality-Adjusted Life-Year
QPP	Quebec Pension Plan, Canada
RCT	randomized controlled trial
RSI	repetitive strain injury
SG	standard gamble
SSDI	Social Security Disability Insurance, United States
TC	total cost
TR	total revenue
VSL	value of a statistical life
WHO	World Health Organization
WTA	willingness to accept
WTP	willingness to pay

Contributors

Benjamin C. Amick III
Institute for Work & Health,
Toronto, Canada

Phil Bigelow
Institute for Work & Health,
Toronto, Canada

Alan Clayton
Australia National University,
National Research Centre for
Occupational Health and Safety
Regulation, Canberra, Australia

Donald C. Cole
Institute for Work & Health,
Toronto, Canada

Richard Cookson
Department of Social Policy,
University of York, Heslington, York,
United Kingdom

Anthony J. Culyer
Department of Economics and
Related Studies,
University of York,
Heslington, York,
United Kingdom

Carolyn S. Dewa
Work and Well-being Research and
Evaluation Program
Centre for Addiction and Mental
Health, Toronto, Canada

Roman Dolinschi
Institute for Work & Health,
Toronto, Canada

Peter Dorman
Department of Environmental
Studies, The Evergreen College,
Olympia, United States

William Gnam
Institute for Work & Health,
Toronto, Canada

Michel Grignon
Departments of Gerontology and
Economics, McMaster University,
Hamilton, Canada

Jeffrey S. Hoch
Centre for Research on Inner City
Health, The Keenan Research Centre
in the Li Ka Shing Knowledge
Institute of St Michael's Hospital,
Toronto, Canada

Ulrike Hotopp
Department for Business, Enterprise
and Regulatory Reform, London,
United Kingdom

Birgit Koeper
Federal Institute for Occupational
Safety and Health (BAuA),
Dortmund, Germany

Thomas Kohstall
Economy and Central Duties
Department, BGAG Institute Work &
Health, Dresden, Germany

Audrey Laporte
Department of Health Policy,
Management and Evaluation, Faculty
of Medicine, University of Toronto,
Toronto, Canada

John Mendeloff
Graduate School of Public
and International Affairs,
University of Pittsburgh, Pittsburgh,
United States

Cameron Mustard
Institute for Work & Health,
Toronto, Canada

Karen Niven
Karen Niven Consulting Ltd.,
Gairneybank, Kinross,
United Kingdom

Claire de Oliveira
Institute for Work & Health,
Toronto, Canada

Lynda Robson
Institute for Work & Health,
Toronto, Canada

Mark Sculpher
Centre for Health Economics,
University of York, Heslington, York,
United Kingdom

Sandra Sinclair
Institute for Work & Health,
Toronto, Canada

Emile Tompa
Institute for Work & Health,
Toronto, Canada

Part 1

Scene setting and context

Chapter 1

The broad conceptualization of work and health

Cameron Mustard

Introduction

Work-related health interventions in industrialized countries have been predominantly concerned with the regulation of materials and processes that are potentially hazardous to the health of workers. Occupational health protection efforts have produced immensely safer, cleaner, and healthier work environments [see Chapter 6 for brief descriptions of the occupational health and safety (OHS) systems in several countries]. Workers' compensation systems in developed economies have frequently used fiscal incentives to influence firm-level practices concerning the prevention and rehabilitation of compensable occupational injuries and diseases. There is evidence that these incentive-based policies are effective instruments for influencing firm behaviour (Hyatt and Thomason 1998).

At the immediate level of the firm, regulation and fiscal incentives are what come to mind when thinking about OHS, and are at the core of many interventions investigated in evaluation studies. However, there is a broader notion of work and health that is of growing interest in many developed countries, one that encapsulates a wide range of exposures and experiences related to the availability and nature of work at a particular point in time, as well as over periods of time.

In this chapter we focus on this broad conceptualization of work and health. We extend the traditional view of occupational health protection to embrace a comprehensive framework of how work may influence health, with a specific focus on the cumulative effects of labour-market experiences over the work career. As depicted in Figure 1.1, we acknowledge the roles of macro-economic factors, labour-market factors and conditions within individual workplaces as being relevant to understand the health consequences of work experiences. We include a brief review of the evidence documenting the biological consequences of adverse psychosocial work experiences and conclude the chapter with a

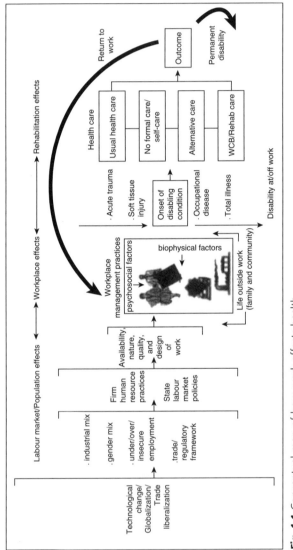

Fig. 1.1 Conceptual map of how work affects health.

consideration of the implications of this evidence for OHS interventions and labour-market policies and practices. This broader conceptualization indicates both that the links between working conditions and health are better understood than hitherto and that new hazards and threats to health are replacing traditional ones. For both reasons evaluation, including economic evaluation, of the options is likely to become both more informative and more urgent.

The burden of occupational injury and disease

Work experiences have pervasive consequences for the health of populations in developed economies. Though annual rates of temporarily disabling occupational morbidity in North America have declined significantly over the past quarter-century, they remain as high as 40 per 1,000 worker-years (Courtney and Webster 1999). In the United States in 2002, the Bureau of Labor Statistics reported 5,524 fatal work injuries, 4.4 million non-fatal injuries and 294,500 illnesses (Schulte 2005). Finnish researchers have estimated that 6.7% of all deaths in Finland in 1996 in ages 25–64 were attributable to occupational factors (Nurminen and Karjalainen 2001). For the United States, Steenland and colleagues (2003) have calculated that 7.4% of deaths (55,200 of 738,000) among people aged 15–69 years in 1997 were from occupational injury and disease. The authors estimated that occupational deaths were the eighth leading cause of death in the United States after diabetes (64,751), and more numerous than motor vehicle accidents (43,501) and suicides (30,573) (Steenland *et al.* 2003).

Schulte (2005) summarized evidence on the risk of mortality, morbidity and injuries attributable to occupational factors in a recent review of 38 studies of the burden of occupational injury and disease. In addition to the well-documented estimate that 15–20% of injuries among working-age adults are attributable to occupational exposures, he estimates the fraction of disease attributed to such exposures. For example, 8–15% of asthma cases and 8–12% of ischaemic heart disease cases among working-age adults may be attributable to occupational exposures.

The accurate attribution of adverse health consequences arising from work has long been recognized as a substantial challenge. Applying conservative assumptions, a number of burden estimates have suggested that occupational injury and disease account for approximately 3% of the total population burden of disability (Leigh *et al.* 1996a; Murray and Lopez 1996). However, these estimates have been criticized for underestimating the true burden of work-related disability, particularly for disease (Driscoll *et al.* 2005; International Labour Organization 2003). For example, Leigh and Robbins (2004) generated estimates of the incidence of occupational disease in the USA from epidemiological studies, and compared these estimates with cases of occupational disease compensated by workers' compensation insurance. Comparisons of the two estimates suggest that in 1999, workers' compensation failed to compensate for 46,000–93,000 deaths (Leigh and Robbins 2004). In earlier work, Kraut (1994) found that a total of 17,290 cases of occupational disease were reported in Canada in 1989, while estimates generated from epidemiological studies suggest the actual incidence of occupational disease was between 57,000–91,000 cases.

The substantial underestimation of occupational disease morbidity and mortality in surveillance estimates based on compensation system records is due to a number of factors. The relationship between work-related exposures and disease processes can be complex. Generally, to establish work-relatedness and compensation eligibility requires evidence that a work exposure led directly to the development of a condition or to a significant exacerbation of a pre-existing condition. However, most diseases have multi-factorial aetiologies (Schulte 2005; Driscoll *et al.* 2005), presenting major theoretical as well as practical problems of attribution in individual cases of disease.

Evidence has accumulated rapidly over the past decade that established causes of work-attributable morbidity represent only the tip of the iceberg of adverse health consequences attributable to work. It is known that common diseases, such as coronary heart disease, mental illness, and degenerative musculoskeletal disease may be initiated or accelerated by chronic adverse work experiences (Marmot and Feeney 1996). There are challenges in documenting the precise contribution of work experiences to the onset and progression of such disorders due to their long latency and multi-factorial nature (Frank and Maetzel 2000). Even more challenging is the identification of effective OHS interventions to address them. However, emerging research evidence distilled from robust longitudinal observational studies in developed countries has increasingly indicated that processes embedded in the experience of work are important causes of the pervasive occupational gradient in life expectancy (Sorlie and Rogot 1990; Kunst *et al.* 1998; Siegrist and Marmot 2004). Essentially, the evidence indicates that workers in low-skilled, low-wage occupations have higher mortality than workers in high-skilled, high-wage occupations, and that there is a gradient rather than a step function relating occupational class to mortality.

Recent prospective studies of young adults entering the labour market have documented the health effects of adverse labour-market experiences (Graetz 1993; Blane *et al.* 1996; Morrell *et al.* 1997; Power and Hertzman 1997; Matthews *et al.* 1998; Wadsworth *et al.* 1999). Work environment characteristics in healthy working adults, such as the degree of control over responses to work demands, have been shown to explain the emergence of occupational

Table 1.1 Total cost (direct and indirect) of occupational injury and disease for selected developed economies.

Country	Base year	Cost as a percent of GDP
Great Britain[1]	1995/96	1.2–1.4
Denmark[1]	1990	2.5
Finland[1]	1992	3.6
Norway[1]	1990	5.6–6.2
Sweden[1]	1990	5.1
Denmark[1]	1992	2.7
Australia [1]	1992/93	3.9
Netherlands[1]	1995	2.6
United States[2]	1992	3.0

Sources: [1]Beatson and Coleman 1997; [2]Leigh et al. 1996b.

morbidity gradients. This remains the case even after adjustments for behavioural risk factors, such as smoking or diet (Bosma *et al.* 1997; Hemingway and Marmot 1999; Borg *et al.* 2000; Mustard *et al.* 2003).

Leigh and colleagues (1996b) estimated that employer costs (represented by insurance premiums) constitute only 11% of the true costs of occupational injury and disease in the United States. Eighty per cent of the true costs are borne by workers and 9% by general taxpayers. These figures suggest that the bulk of the economic costs of occupational injuries and diseases are externalized. This has important implications for undertaking comprehensive economic evaluations, since using workers compensation claims data and taking a firm perspective will capture only a small subset of the total costs and consequences. Table 1.1 reports estimates of the direct and indirect costs of occupational injury and disease in a sample of developed economies. In general, the average financial burden approaches 3% of gross domestic product.

Documenting the biological consequences of adverse work experiences

The evidence linking specific experiences in the labour market to physiological response and, in turn, to altered states of metabolism, physiology, or immune function were assessed in a systematic review by Lavis *et al.* (1998). The studies selected for inclusion were restricted to prospective observational designs where exposure to labour-market experiences preceded the measurement of health outcomes. Selected studies concentrated on the assessment of the health effects of unemployment, job insecurity, job characteristics, and job position within the firm. Studies of the impact of unemployment have focused on cortisol, serum cholesterol levels, blood pressure, and lymphocyte reactivity, and have found evidence of altered regulatory function following unemployment (Lavis *et al.* 1998). Although Lavis and colleagues (1998) found no studies linking unemployment to the initiation or progression of diseases, they identified a large body of work that had consistently found the experience of unemployment to be associated with a heightened risk of death in the period following the unemployment spell.

With regard to the nature of work, a body of literature has identified a strong and consistent association between job characteristics, such as decision latitude, and disease incidence (especially cardiovascular disease), as well as between job position in the firm and disease risk. Lavis and colleagues (1998), for example, examined the relationship between job demands, job control, and physiology, including blood pressure, serum cholesterol levels, and pro-lactin. In examining the role of the nature of work on disease initiation and progression, Brunner (1996) focused on cardiovascular disease and the related cluster of features known as the metabolic syndrome (central adiposity, elevated insulin, high blood pressure and elevated serum cortisol levels). The predominant finding has been that individuals chronically exposed to adverse psychosocial working environments have an elevated risk both of cardiovascular disease and mortality attributable to it (Bosma *et al.* 1998; Hemingway and Marmot 1999; Belkic *et al.* 2004). Although these findings are based on observational research designs, they appear robust in that the studies have generally achieved adequate measurement of potential confounders and do not appear to be due to the differential distribution of health behaviours in occupational groups.

Jobs characterized by adverse psychosocial conditions are not randomly distributed throughout the occupational hierarchy. High-status occupations, which have professional-level entry criteria and relatively high compensation, are most commonly characterized by high levels of demands and responsibili-ties. At the same time, there are also high levels of latitude, control, and auton-omy for responding to the demands. In contrast, many low-status occupations, especially those associated with machine-paced production or scheduled per-formance requirements, are characterized by a combination of high demands and limited discretionary autonomy to respond to them. There is increasing evidence that the distribution of these job characteristics across the occupa-tional hierarchy is among the factors accounting for the distribution of cardiovascular risk factors and related cardiovascular disease mortality in working-age populations (Belkic *et al.* 2000).

Several cohort studies have also documented the emergence of occupational hierarchy-related health status gradients associated with the work exposures. In a study of Danish workers who had reported good health at baseline, differential exposure to adverse psychosocial job characteristics was related to the risk of reporting a decline in perceived health status over a five-year follow-up period (Borg *et al.* 2000). The study found that the results were not attributable to other potential explanatory factors such as differences in health behaviours amongst members of different occupational groups. Similar results have been replicated in cohorts in other Organization for Economic Cooperation and Development (OECD) countries (Martikainen *et al.* 1999; Mustard *et al.* 2003).

Changes in the nature of work

Over the past 25 years, developed economies have experienced significant changes in the structure of labour markets and in the organization of work. A dramatic shift in the sectoral distribution of employment has been among the most profound changes of developed economies over this period. The shift is reminiscent of the equally sharp changes that occurred as labour moved from farms to factories in the first quarter of the twentieth century (Reich 1996; Rifkin 1996). From the 1970s to the early 1990s the proportion of the labour force employed in manufacturing fell and the proportion employed in the service sector rose, such that by 1991, 78% of the Group of Seven countries' workforce were employed in services (Daniels 1993; Castells and Aoyama 1994).

Along with changes in the sectoral distribution of employment, several related structural trends have occurred within occupations. During the past two decades, there has been an overall upgrading in the skill level required for jobs in the United States (Howell and Wolff 1991), Canada (Myles 1988; Livingstone 1999), and the United Kingdom (Gallie 2000). Among British workers asked about their perception of skill requirements changes from 1981 to 1992, 26.2% reported an increase in the skill requirements for their job (Gallie 2000). The highest proportion of workers reporting increased skill requirements was among the semi- and unskilled manual occupational categories. In the absence of other changes in the nature of work, increases in skill requirements would be expected to be translated into higher earnings and, potentially, into higher job satisfaction. There is evidence of a substantial paradox that has emerged in labour markets over the past two decades, in which increasing worker productivity has become disconnected from the earnings received by workers (Palley 1998).

In addition to increased skill requirements within jobs, there has been a trend toward increasing entry requirements independently of actual skill requirements (a trend known as credential inflation), particularly for unskilled jobs (Holzer 1996; Livingstone 1999). For example, in a large study of Ontario workers, Holzer (1996) compared the qualifications required for various occupations in the early 1980s and the mid-1990s. He found that the requirement for postsecondary education in unskilled manual and clerical occupations increased by 60 and 96%, respectively, compared with a decrease of 3% for managerial occupations and an increase of 6% for professional jobs. These somewhat high rates of credential inflation for unskilled workers are one example of the labour-market transformations that have altered the availability of work in low-skilled occupations.

The labour-market changes during the last quarter of a century have occurred against a backdrop of historically high unemployment (Hobsbawm 1994). In the United States, annual average unemployment rates from 1973 to the early 1990s generally were at least 2% higher than the rates from 1947 to 1973 (Mishel *et al.* 1997). In OECD nations, unemployment rates during the 1980s were approximately double those of the 1970s (Navarro 2001).

Persistently high unemployment has also contributed to a pervasive sense of employment insecurity among workers. Between the 1970s and the 1990s, job insecurity (measured on a six-point scale ranging from secure to insecure jobs) increased from 3.5 to 4.5 or 1.5 standard deviations (Karasek *et al.* 1998). The eroding norm of long-term employment engagement, the declining influence of organized labour in defining the nature of work, and an ascendancy of shareholders' interests in corporate governance, have increased workers' exposure to the risk of layoff. Median job tenure has also declined over this period. For example, throughout the economic expansion of the 1990s, the annual proportion of USA workers experiencing dislocation increased from 8% to more than 12% of the labour force (Osterman 1999). Although some of this increase in employment insecurity may have been cyclical, there has been an increased turbulence in the labour market even during periods of economic expansion, particularly for lower-paid and lower-quality occupations.

Another major trend in labour-market dynamics over the past quarter-century in Europe, North America, and Australia, has been a rise in non-standard work arrangements, such as part-time work, shift work, self-employment, multiple job holding, and casual or temporary work (Quinlan 1998; Quinlan *et al.* 2001). These new, flexible labour arrangements have been evident across many economic sectors. The increase in part-time employment has been particularly marked. In 1953, 3.8% of the Canadian workforce was employed part-time. By 1980, this had risen to 13.5% and by 1993, to 17.3% (Duffy *et al.* 1997). By 1989, the share of the Swedish workforce employed part-time was 24%; in the United Kingdom it was 22%; and in Japan and the United States it was 18% (Livingstone 1999). Increases in part-time employment have gone hand in hand with increases in multiple job holding. During the 1980s in Canada, the number of female multiple-job holders increased by 89% (28% among males; Duffy and Pupo 1992).

Although the emergence of non-standard work arrangements is a visible example of the structural changes in the nature of work in developed economies, the proportion of the labour force in employment arrangements that are formally insecure (i.e., limited in the duration of employment) is relatively small. Fewer than 10% of USA workers are in contract, on-call, or temporary agency employment (Osterman 1999). There is also good evidence that the growth in these forms of employment, which are also called contingent work, levelled off in the 1990s in the United States (Osterman 1999).

In addition to declines in the security of employment arrangements, there have been important changes in the organization of work within firms in many economic sectors. In particular, management hierarchies have flattened in many service and manufacturing industries as employers adopted models of high-performance work organizations (Osterman 1999). Evidence suggests that the prevalence of job strain and work intensity has increased in workplaces in the United States and in some European countries (Landsbergis et al. 1999). European surveys have shown that the proportion of high-strain jobs (i.e., work with low control, low support, and high demands) increased from 25 to 30% between 1991 and 1996 (European Foundation 1997; Bond et al. 1998). From 1990 to 2000, three waves of the European Survey on Working Conditions documented increases in the pace and intensity of work, especially among white-collar workers (Paoli and Merllie 2001). The monitoring of changes over time in the organization of work has produced an uneven portrait. There is disquieting evidence of decline in the quality of many occupational roles and in a range of working conditions, despite evidence of new organizational practices with the potential to improve the quality of working life (Lowe 2000).

Policies to improve work environments

With the exception of Scandinavian countries, governments and employers have given little concerted attention to reducing adverse exposures related to the nature and availability of work. There are perhaps three principal explanations for this lack of policy commitment. First, the scientific evidence for the causal attribution of chronic cardiovascular, musculoskeletal, and mental health disorders to psychosocial work conditions and labour-market experiences has emerged only in the past decade (Hemingway and Marmot 1999). Furthermore, the evidence that the disorders in question are inherently multifactorial and, therefore, only partially attributable to work experiences has complicated policy-related decision making (Frank and Maetzel 2000). Secondly, the implications of this evidence for modifications to work processes and work organization impinge directly on the principle, strongly held by employers, that firms should retain considerable autonomy in setting work processes and environments. Regulatory efforts to impose constraints on this autonomy have been aggressively contested in most jurisdictions (Hoover 2000). Thirdly, government regulation of labour-market practices concerning the rights and duties of employers and workers, hours of work, and employment insurance and pension systems have not traditionally incorporated a prominent health-impact perspective.

Notwithstanding this history, clear opportunities exist to improve the health of working-age populations through improvements in work environments. Active labour-market policies focused on modifying work environments might productively focus on three areas: research and monitoring, regulatory actions, and economic incentives for the employer.

Ongoing research efforts are needed regarding the magnitude of health effects associated with working conditions and labour-market experiences. In addition, it is necessary to monitor adverse labour-market experiences both at the population/workforce level and the work organization level (Smulders *et al.* 1996; Lavis *et al.* 2001).

Regulatory intervention, with a focus on reform and innovation in the institutional structure of the labour market, may be needed to redress the significant shift over the past quarter-century toward greater employer versus worker authority in determining factors such as the quality of working conditions and employment security. There is growing evidence that mandatory joint management-labour mechanisms can effectively improve both the health and productivity of the work environment (Theorell 1999; Kompier and Cooper 1999; O'Grady 2000). The growth of non-standard employment and the decline in union membership (particularly in the private sector) can be expected to weaken the effectiveness of joint management–labour mechanisms. In this context, policy actions designed to strengthen joint governance authority in firms and across economic sectors would contribute to halting the deterioration in working conditions that have implications for the health of the workforce. Regulation will also continue to be important in defining limits to the biomechanical and psychosocial intensity of work.

Policy initiatives are not keeping pace with research evidence that has clarified the long-term health effects of cumulative exposure to adverse psychosocial work environments. Policy initiatives also need to address the structuring of reward and deterrence incentives to signal desirable employment practices to firms. Policymakers may draw lessons from the workers' compensation system practices regarding insurance premiums which are now broadly applied in North America and Europe. These practices provide premium reductions to firms with low injury rates and charge higher premiums to firms with high injury rates. It may be useful to consider extending such firm-level incentives to other payroll tax instruments. For example, firms with high rates of employment dislocation over time could be charged premium supplements on employment insurance premiums that recognize the short-term health care costs associated with unemployment (Betcherman 1995; Kraut *et al.* 2000). On a longer time horizon, a similar mechanism could be explored to set differential firm premiums in universal pension and health insurance programmes to anticipate higher or lower rates of work disability arising from firm-level work organization practices.

Conclusion

In the developed economies, people rank work experiences as being among the most rewarding aspects of their lives. However, labour-market experiences can lead workers to be exposed to hazardous physical or chemical environments or adverse psychosocial work environments that have substantial risks to health.

This chapter has reviewed the well-documented burden of ill health in working age populations attributable to work experiences, both the traditional concerns of OHS and more recent concerns regarding adverse psychosocial working conditions. There is convincing evidence that the burden of occupational injury and disease is underestimated in regular occupational health surveillance systems.

The health implications of labour-market changes that have occurred over the past quarter century can be summarized in four dimensions. First, work clearly has become safer, both as a result of regulatory actions to reduce exposures to physical and chemical hazards, and as a result of the replacement of human labour with machines made possible by advances in technology.

Second, as global economic integration has altered the demand for labour in regional economies, instability in the availability of work in many sectors of the developed economies has increased. Many traditional sectors have contracted, whereas the service sector has expanded. This churning of the labour market has been associated with higher rates of employment dislocation, shorter median work tenure, longer duration of unemployment spells, and the growth of insecure work arrangements in the formal wage economy. Health consequences from an increasingly insecure labour market may arise as a result of income insecurity and, simultaneously, as a result of the cumulative effects of physiological responses to the perception of insecurity or the experience of job dislocation.

Third, labour-market changes have altered the nature of work in many industries. With the reduction of demand for low-skilled occupations and pressures to increase productivity, evidence has emerged that some sectors have experienced increased intensification of work and prevalence of high-strain work environments (Ostry *et al.* 2000; Woodward *et al.* 1999). From both a biomechanical and a physiological perspective, an optimal evolution of work environments would entail a reduction, rather than an increase, in these potentially adverse exposures.

Lastly, the reduction in demand for low-skilled occupations has led to a stagnation of market earnings among those workers, contributing to a growing inequality in earnings for workers in developed economies. The proportion of workers whose labour-market income is below a minimally adequate level is increasing, rather than decreasing. For example, the real value of the US minimum wage declined from 117% of the three-person family poverty threshold in 1968 to 80% of the threshold in 1998 (Pollin and Luce 1998). The health effects of poverty are well documented. It is a paradox, indicative of market failure, that a sustained period of economic growth over the past 25 years has produced an increase in the number of people whose labour-market income is below a minimum level of adequacy. The greatest risk of exposure to adverse working experiences has traditionally been associated with lower-status occupations, and the evidence summarized here indicates that both the availability of work and the nature of work have deteriorated over the past two decades among persons in these occupations. The magnitude of these changes in the nature and availability of work is sufficiently large to raise concerns for the short-term and long-term health consequences for the working-age population.

Active labour-market policies can address these changes, and there is ample evidence of effective instruments available to the state to mitigate the adverse health consequences of the contemporary labour market. Optimal labour-market policy would find an appropriate balance amongst the interests of corporations, workers, and society at large, and the health effects of labour-market experiences should be an important part of the policymaking calculus. However, policies appear to have become increasingly neglectful of worker health effects. The evidence presented in this chapter argues for more accounting of the health consequences of labour-market experiences in informing labour-market policy decisions and workplace policies and practices.

Chapter 2

What is a little more health and safety worth?

Anthony J. Culyer, Benjamin C. Amick III, and
Audrey Laporte

Introduction

In this chapter we introduce readers to the principal ways in which economists
evaluate workplace health and safety investments. We draw extensively on
work that has been done in the field of health care, although there are major
differences and challenges posed by the analysis of workplace interventions for
health and safety that are largely absent in the field of health care. Our main
intention is to prepare the ground for subsequent chapters on specific issues
by opening up for explicit consideration the following fundamental questions:

- Is safety an end or a means to other ends, such as better health and
  uninterrupted earnings?

- Ought better health be the ultimate objective of workplace interventions,
  or ought improved productivity, lower insurance payouts, and lower
  insurance premiums be considered as important?

- Why is a focus on regulation and control sometimes preferred to reliance
  on market forces in generating desirable changes in workplace health and
  safety?

- What key value judgments are involved in evaluating workplace health and
  safety policies, and who ought to be making them?

- To what philosophical tradition does the economic approach belong?

- Is economic analysis undertaken in order to discover what is best for
  society or to predict what is likely to happen as a consequence of particular
  actions?

- How can analysts remain scientific while at the same time addressing
  questions such as 'what is best for society' that are inherently value-laden?

- What *is* a little more health and safety worth?

The innocent-sounding question posed in the title of this chapter is our way into these issues. It is meant to lead us into an exploration of the issues that arise in evaluating the effectiveness and cost-effectiveness of workplace interventions to promote health and safety (note that some researchers may consider that cost-effectiveness already includes effectiveness, but it is a distinction commonly made and familiar to many people (see Box 2.1 for some basic definitions)).

Ends and means

Our thesis question may appear odd to those in the world of workplace health and safety who are not economists. After all, better health seems a reasonable objective for individuals and governments to aim at. It is an end, but safety at work is a means—one of many—to the end of better health. More precisely, the means are the methods by which risks to health in the workplace are managed; so the means are the instruments, policies, workplace interventions, and the like, that are adopted in workplaces and reduce the probabilities of events occurring which are harmful to health. These means are at best intermediate outcomes that lie on the road to the more ultimate outcome, better health. Hence, the worthiness of any risk reduction is presumably to be

---

Box 2.1 Some basic definitions

Efficacy, effectiveness, and cost-effectiveness

Efficacy: the positive impact on health and other outcomes of an intervention when it is performed under ideal conditions, such as in a randomized controlled trial when full adherence is ensured.

Effectiveness: the positive impact on health and other outcomes of an intervention when it is performed under usual operating conditions.

Cost-effectiveness: the effect on health and other outcomes of an intervention subject to a limit on the available resources for its implementation or, equivalently, the resource cost necessary to achieve a given effect on health and other outcomes, usually relative to some alternative, such as the status quo or a rival intervention.

Cost-effectiveness analysis: the systematic consideration of the effect on health and other outcomes of an intervention relative to the resources used for its implementation, usually evaluated through a comparison with some alternative, such as the status quo or a rival intervention.

measured in terms of its impact on health. Considering the value both of health and safety is to invite the danger of double counting (see Box 2.2 on forms of double counting). It is health that is to be valued. The value of safety depends primarily on the value of the incremental health it enables.

However, means and ends can become intertwined. Less risk, independent of any health or other consequences, may be preferred since people are generally risk-averse. Just feeling more secure is a benefit. It is not a health benefit in the conventional sense of what health is, but it does affect a person's welfare.

One might focus on consequences other than health. For example, an employer may implement engineering controls in order to eliminate a safety hazard and increase productivity without considering the direct value of health benefits. This suggests another perspective, one that does not view health as the ultimate objective, but rather increased productivity. From such a perspective the means remain the reductions in risk, but the end is increased output, something to which it is relatively easy to attach a monetary value. Of course, in many cases health and safety interventions enhance both health and productivity.

Notwithstanding the fact that safety is in many cases a means, we have identified three ends associated with resource investment in health and safety that are of value to society: improved health, the inherent value of greater security, and enhanced productivity. Resource use may be directly linked to improved health, as is the case with health care services. In some cases productivity effects

Box 2.2 Forms of double counting

Double counting is a hazard in any method of appraising options. There are three common forms:

Simple errors: due to incorrect arithmetic.

Suspicious circumstances: due to fraudulent accounting practices.

Subtler forms: due to poor administrative records or poor accounting of resource costs.

Example 1: logging a medical procedure in two places even though it was performed only once, due to the patient being transferred from one hospital to another at some stage, while the procedure was being undertaken.

Example 2: computing and adding the cost of a surgeon's time for an operation when that cost is already included in the total fee.

Example 3: adding increased earnings effects to the consequences even though they have already been included in a patient-based measure of the increase in the quality of life.

(note that we use the terms 'consequence', 'benefit', and 'effect' interchangeably) may arise through the impact of resources on health, as when effective disability management enables a safe return to work sooner than would otherwise have been the case or when sickness absences are reduced through safer working conditions. In other cases, productivity may be affected directly through workplace safety enhancements. There may also be a link from productivity increases to health increases. These various pathways are depicted in Figure 2.1 below.

Two types of complexity are involved in the foregoing. The first is a complexity arising out of the need to determine what consequences ought to be considered. Three beneficial consequences have been mentioned and depicted in the diagram, but what other possible candidates are there and how are they to be measured and compared? Furthermore, consequences to whom? Is it only those to workers, or ought we also to consider workers' families and dependents, owners of firms, insurance agencies, and consumers of the outputs produced by the workplaces in question? When we use the word 'ought,' what are the ethical criteria to which we are appealing? These are lofty questions, which we try to address in what follows in this chapter. The second complexity concerns the pathways of causation and interaction between means and ends, and how some ends can even, as we have seen, in turn become means.

These complexities are familiar challenges to economists. The first set involves a discussion of human welfare, its measurement, distribution, and aggregation. The second involves the production function or, in other words, the analysis of the ways in which inputs are transformed into outputs and how feedback effects are taken into account.

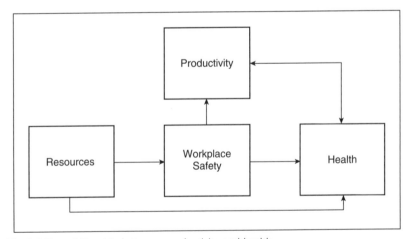

Fig. 2.1 The relationship between productivity and health.

Cost-effectiveness analysis (CEA) is something of a hybrid of the two kinds of complexity. It usually considers both benefits and opportunity costs as being dependent on people's preferences and it tends to be action-orientated by focusing on the use of technologies to change workplace practices or on the technologies of health care. The notion of technology can be very broad: a drug, a guard on a machine, non-slip surfaces, an OHS management system, a modification to a health insurance system such as the introduction of a no-fault system, or the introduction of experience-rated employers' premiums. In effect, the technologies that are evaluated in cost-effectiveness analysis are 'ways of doing things'.

The philosophical framing of economic evaluation

The approach economists generally adopt is known as 'consequentialism' in philosophical writing. Consequentialism is a class of ethical theories sharing the view that the morality of actions or arrangements is to be judged by their consequences. Consequentialism is often contrasted with deontological moral theories, which hold that the morality of actions and arrangements is to be judged in terms of duties and rights. Essentially, consequentialism is the notion that the outcome ought to justify the means. The most famous approach within this class is called 'act utilitarianism' (see Box 2.3).

Consequentialism may not be a useful approach in some decision contexts. For example, considering only costs and consequences is certainly not the only way of evaluating the pros and cons of alternatives for a disciplinary case. One may want to take account of the motives of a person who might be subject to disciplinary action. There are other objections to consequentialism. The most common one comes in the form of a dogmatic statement, 'the end can never justify the means', but if an end cannot justify a means, then what can? It may be that a particular end does not justify a particular means, and it may also be that some means are so awful that they cannot be justified by any end, but, if there is a justification for adopting any particular means of advancing safety at work, we adopt the working hypothesis that it lies in its consequences for workers' health, for their families' welfare, for productivity, for the need for compensation and, indeed, for the well-being of any and all those affected by it.

The question of perspective

There is a value judgment in the foregoing. We have asserted that the justification ought to be in terms of the well-being of any and all who are affected by it. This is to adopt a particular perspective, commonly termed the 'societal perspective'. In the world of affairs this is not always and perhaps

Box 2.3 Utility theories

What is utility in economics

Utility in economics is an abstract way of ordering a person's preferences by assigning numbers to the consumption of goods and services, or to characteristics of goods and services. It can be measured either as an ordinal (like temperature) or a cardinal (like distance) construct.

Ethical theories based on utilitarianism

The three most common theories based on utilitarianism are:

Act utilitarianism: the right thing to do is any action that generates, on balance, the most utility.

Preference utilitarianism: the right thing to do is whatever best matches the preferences (utilities) of the people who are deemed to count in society.

Rule utilitarianism: the right thing to do is to follow the rule that is most likely to generate the most utility, if it were generally to be followed.

rarely the way in which decisions are reached. In some workplaces, the decisions will be taken by managers who see their prime responsibility as being to serve the interests of owners, so that interventions having benefits that accrue exclusively to workers will not gain acceptance. Workers, on the other hand, may perceive only the benefits that accrue to them, fight to achieve them, and ignore the disadvantages that fall on the owners. Plainly, the distribution of costs and consequences affects behaviour, attitudes, and the chances of success in advocacy. In practical politics these things matter. But they also matter when a deeper ethical question is addressed: 'what policies, controls, regulations, interventions, inspections, penalties and rewards and the like ought to be introduced?' Or put another way: 'what is the value of a little more safety in the workplace, and of value to whom?'

Another notable feature of the question in the title of this chapter is that it needs to be asked at all. One might have expected that the question of the worthwhileness of health and safety would have been resolved long ago, or at least that the methods by which an answer is to be reached, and the principles underlying those methods, would have been long-since settled.

The answer may lie partly in the inherent difficulty of conceptualizing and measuring the effects of workplace health and safety interventions.

Conducting experiments that control for confounders in hugely complex work situations is virtually impossible. Another part of the answer lies, we conjecture, in the way that the academic disciplines that are closely engaged in the OHS field have been applied. It seems that many analysts amongst the practitioners of the various clinical, statistical, public health and social scientific fields engaged with workplace health and safety issues view more health and better safety as always preferred, regardless of what they may cost. It is really only a question of figuring out what works. There has been, we detect, a tendency to see things through the lenses of the workers. Moreover, scientists have often not set out to refute hypotheses about the effectiveness of the means they adopt or recommend, but rather have focused on proving them, thus reversing the standard scientific and statistical approach to hypothesis testing (we are not intending to imply support for naïve falsification here). In opposition are views that may be more characteristic of employers, for whom the lens of worker welfare may seem less relevant, unless there were some indirect effects on profitability, and for whom the bottom line and managerial convenience may be the dominant considerations. Neither set of attitudes is to be despised, but a truly analytical approach to addressing the question of the social value of greater workplace safety and better worker health must find some way of escaping sectional bias.

Scylla, Charybdis, and a safe passage

There are three commonly used approaches to evaluating health and safety procedures. Navigating around the first two, we feel much like Odysseus sailing around Scylla and Charybdis, the rocky reef and whirlpool in the straits of Messina. In what follows, we outline each of the three approaches, explain the disadvantages of the first two, and describe our reasons for preferring the third. The three go by the following names: the perfect market approach, the human capital approach and the decision-maker approach.

The perfect market approach

The perfect market approach is premised on the notion that markets function reasonably efficiently, thus rendering formal evaluation of the effectiveness of health and safety procedures unnecessary. The general objective and ultimate criterion for deciding 'worthwhileness' embodied in this approach is the standard economic maximand: the sum of the expected utilities of all affected persons. This leads one to the Panglossian conclusion that the world is best left as it is (Dr Pangloss was Candide's mentor, for whom the world today was the best of all possible worlds). Workers and employers are best left free to negotiate mutually agreeable terms of employment, which cover wages, salaries, other benefits, and workplace safety. Both sides can shop around without incurring any costs, according to their preferences and, in particular, their attitudes towards risk, in order to find a suitable matching of person to job and job environment. Those who are risk-averse will seek safe environments or require compensation for working in riskier workplaces, and trade off the positive and negative aspects of the various offers of labour or employment available. All other things being equal, safer environments will tend to be associated with higher priced products and lower real wages than less safe environments, as there will be no necessity for employers with safer environments to offer compensating wage differentials. In equilibrium, all pros and cons will have been duly weighed within the overall resource constraints of the economy and safety and health will have been optimized, along with everything else.

In such a vision of the world, neither the interventionist policies we commonly observe, nor the normative economic calculations that can underpin them, are necessary. Nor even are voluntary collective actions by firms such as the Voluntary Protection Programs in the US (Rees 1988). A risk that is voluntarily adopted after whatever compensation is agreeable to the consenting parties is a socially acceptable risk. It is the best that can be done in a world in which risk of injury and disease is generally to be avoided, but is, in practice, costly to avoid.

In general, the theory of compensating wage differentials predicts that jobs requiring a higher level of education will, other things equal, pay more than those requiring a lower education in order to compensate employees for their investment in additional education. Jobs associated with higher risk of injury or disease will, other things equal, pay risk-averse workers more than they could earn in other safer jobs for which they are qualified, thus compensating them for the greater likelihood that their working life may be shortened, as well as for any financial and psychic costs they might suffer due to injury or disease.

Compensating wage differentials must be offered by employers who save on health and safety costs by offering less desirable work environments. Such differentials enable unpleasant, but necessary, jobs to be done. Employers who improve the health and safety of work environments do not have to offer compensating wage differentials, but they incur the costs of the improved work environments. Whether environmental changes at work dominate over wage adjustments will depend partly on the relative costs to the employer of changing work environments, and the anticipated responses of potential workers to these changes and any changes in pecuniary offers.

The extent to which markets generate the desired results depends on the efficiency of the matching process between workers and jobs in the economy. John Stuart Mill, the great utilitarian, observed at the turn of the twentieth century that there were imperfections in the market which often resulted in the least pleasant jobs also paying the lowest wages under circumstances which could only implausibly be interpreted as offering a net compensating advantage of any kind (Mill 1965). He also noted that significant unemployment would constrain workers' ability to negotiate higher wages or to reject job offers. Mill further argued that people from marginalized groups, such as immigrants, or poor and ill-educated people, could be ghettoized into the least desired employment strata within the labour market, leading to an over-supply of such people in competition for the least desirable jobs.

The compensating wage differential model assumes free and complete information on the part of workers and employers. However, if workers are unable to assess the risk of injury or disease accurately, they may not negotiate a sufficiently high wage. While there is some evidence to suggest that workers are fairly good at assessing risk of death, they are less able to assess the risk of chronic disease, or acute events, such as injury arising from slips and trips on shop floors (Dorman 1996). Supervisory and work-group relationships may lead workers systematically to over- or underestimate the significance of the various job attributes. While workers might, over time, acquire a good perception of the bundle of job characteristics, the threat of moving to another position if wage compensation or other adjustments in the package were not implemented may be weakened, and this weakness can be reinforced if health, pension, seniority, and other benefits are at risk of being lost. Hence, the high costs of changing jobs can impede the effective working of the market mechanism. High rates of staff turnover are also costly to employers, since they may lose workers in whose skills they have invested. They will also incur hiring costs and may incur short-term losses in productivity.

Externalities are another source of market imperfection (see Box 2.4 for a definition) Many aspects of working conditions are external to the decision makers in that they affect third parties either financially, physically or psychically. For example, Leigh *et al.* (1996) estimated that workers' compensation insurance premiums paid by employers represent only 11% of the costs of occupational injury and disease in the United States; the remainder of the costs fall to workers and taxpayers. The total economic burden is estimated at around 3% of Gross Domestic Product, but only 10% of this burden is borne directly by employers. When external costs are added to internal costs, it amounts to what economists call 'social cost'. Yet it does not follow that the activity that generates external costs ought to be eliminated, nor does it follow that externalities should be eliminated should there be ways of reducing them.

The optimal social adjustment will be one that induces the firm to act as though it recognized the external cost so as to reduce the activity rate to that at

Box 2.4 Externalities

'Externality' is an economics term for the effects on others of a person's or group's decisions. These effects can be both positive and negative. Economists classify costs as internal (i.e., those that fall on the decision maker, such as wages and salaries) and external (i.e., those that fall on others, such as the smoke of a factory that pollutes the air in a community and burdens it with increased cleaning costs, disease, etc.). The sum of internal and external costs is called social cost. Similarly, benefits may be internal, such as the revenue from sales, or external, such as the blossoms of a farmer's orchard that is made available to the bees in a nearby honey farm.

There are three basic types of externality:

Pecuniary externalities: affect the value of other resources, as when an innovation makes unskilled labour redundant or increases the value of skilled labour.

Physical externalities: affect the physical characteristics of other people or their property, as in the case of disease communicated via workplaces, or as herd immunity is acquired through vaccination.

Utility or psychic externalities: affect the sensibilities of others, as when the knowledge of poor working conditions of some people makes one feel wretched, or the knowledge of good employment practices makes one glad.

which the marginal social benefit equals the marginal social cost. In the case of reducing the externality by other methods, the principle is again that the optimal investment is that at which the social cost of reducing the risk of harmful events is set equal to the best estimate of the social benefit from it, i.e., the benefit to workers plus that accruing to the externally affected parties.

The important logical implication of this is that, because there is a cost to reducing harm, it will generally be the case that there is an optimal degree of reduced harm, which falls short of complete elimination. Economic analysis treats the benefits from hazard reduction in the same way as it treats other benefits. The art, therefore, lies in judging the point at which reducing a hazard costs more than the reduction is considered to be worth. This leads us to the critical issue of perspective. One needs to consider whose costs and benefits matter. In turn, this leads us to the issue of distributive justice or equity, a topic we return to later.

The absence of full employment, imperfect information, lack of perfect labour mobility across jobs, and the existence of externalities suggests that the market, left to its own devices, will *not* yield an optimal level of compensation for risk and, therefore, workers will face a higher than optimal level of risk. This discrepancy provides the basic case for government intervention through workplace health and safety regulation, imposition of minimum OHS standards, education and public information programmes, and evaluative research including the use of analytical methods of assessing risks to health, the social significance of such risks to employers, workers, their families, and the wider community, the availability of technologies through which such risks might be reduced, the costs of implementing such technologies, and the distribution of those costs across employers, employees and the wider community.

There is also the issue of equity, which is related to the fairness of the initial distribution of wealth and power and the advantages and disadvantages that result to various players in the labour market. Many social inequities are multiple. Health is systematically correlated with wealth, as it is to income. In general, the least well-off financially are also the least healthy and well-educated. They are also often the least empowered and organized. Regulatory and other interventions have often been applied on these grounds alone, regardless of the foregoing efficiency considerations outlined in this section. So even if the market actually was perfect, its outcome may well not be regarded as equitable. Those most at risk would in general be the poorest paid, the least skilled, and least educated. The pay-off to investment in safety as seen by managers would rise in proportion to the productivity of the employees most affected, so safety investments that benefited the rich would dominate over those that benefited the poor. Such an outcome would violate the most basic principles of horizontal and vertical equity: that people who are alike in relevant respects ought to be treated alike and those who are not alike in relevant respects ought to be treated unequally in relation to their relevant differences. That is, unless one is prepared to argue that productivity differentials are morally relevant aspects that justify such discrimination.

Dismissing the perfect market line of thought will tend to also require dismissing benefit estimation techniques based on market behaviour. This is particularly the case in cost–benefit studies that use estimates of, for example, willingness to pay for reductions in risk of injury or death (e.g., Moore and Viscusi 1988; Gegax *et al.* 1991), or that use observed wage differentials across employments judged to be similar in most respects, except for the risks to which they expose workers, in order to estimate the cost of safety (e.g., Rosen 1986; Knieser and Leeth 1991). These are vulnerable to the same criticisms on the grounds both of efficiency and equity. The occasions when they are sufficiently immune to such objections always need careful assessment. In general, we think that the usual presumption has to be that the distortions are large and significant. So it is the use of market-based, benefit estimation techniques, rather than their rejection, that needs explicit justification on a case by case basis.

That was our Scylla. If it can be skilfully sailed around, the would-be evaluator is likely to be confronted by our Charybdis: the human capital approach.

The human capital approach

The human capital approach dates back to the earliest attempts at applied economics with William Petty (1899) and William Farr (1853). Petty discounted estimated wages to infinity to compute a capital value, while Farr discounted the difference between future income and an estimated cost of future maintenance, adjusted for the probability of death (for details on discounting see Chapter 12). That, essentially, is the approach adopted today by those using the human capital approach, such as Health Canada (1998). It is, to put things rather sharply, tantamount to treating humans as though they were carthorses. They are good only for what they produce, after deducting what they cost in fodder and watering (for details on this criticism, see Pritchard and Sculpher 2000). The approach neglects any benefit to individuals that is not work-related, as for example, the direct benefit of being free from pain, or not depressed, or not severely stressed, or able to move about. It neglects the value to individuals of leisure time and it also fails to consider any external valuations of people's time, such as valuations by their families and friends.

The method is particularly vulnerable to equity objections. If one person's human capital is worth twice that of another, then it will be worth expending twice as much to avoid losing a certain fraction of it. So those who have expectation of monetarily productive life will have further benefits heaped upon them in the shape of safer workplaces and better rehabilitation.

Of further detriment to the approach is that it is not grounded in any modern welfare economics theory. The conventional neoclassical position is that the appropriate valuation of a reduction in the probability of loss of life is a person's willingness to pay for such a reduction. Although subject to the same objections on the grounds of equity as the perfect market method, it is less susceptible to the efficiency objections provided that the willingness to pay can be obtained under appropriately controlled experimental conditions and provided that external effects are taken into account (Jones-Lee 1989; Jones-Lee *et al.* 1985). The obvious alternative to willingness to pay to avoid a harm is willingness to be compensated for accepting it, but this too is not captured by the human capital approach.

Matters become more complicated if the maximand is more comprehensive. For example, estimates of the benefits over a working lifetime of a workplace safety intervention will underestimate the total productive value of a life by assigning a zero worth to childhood and retirement. If averted productivity losses are simply added to other types of estimates, such as averted losses of health and the averted costs of health care, there is the risk of serious double counting. Depending on the construction of a health outcome measure, the value of work and its contribution to one's standard of living over time will already be embodied in the measure. If already included, the only productivity component that ought to be added is the friction cost associated with replacing a worker such as delays in replacement, cost of recruitment and training. (Koopmanschap *et al.* 1995; Koopmanschap and Rutten 1996; see also Chapter 11).

Does the difference matter? The difference in question is that between treating people as carthorses, on the one hand, and as intelligent people (not mere consumers either), on the other. The issue arises from the fact that humans are both factors of production and also sentient beings. In some cases public policy emphasizes the productive role of people, while in others it emphasizes their human characteristics. The tension in public policy arises from the fact that the best estimate of benefit that the human capital approach can hope to achieve is a precise measure of the market productivity of workers. The best to be hoped for from an alternative based on an evaluation of the consequences for the quality of a person's life, is a set of relevant and believable measures of characteristics of people and their working environments—features that are not directly marketed at all. Those characteristics are essentially health and safety. Health services are marketed, and so are goods and services that contribute to safety, but health and safety as such are not. They are like the environmental characteristics of societies that are not marketed even though they have impact on the prices of assets such as houses (e.g., pollution, noisiness, and beautiful views). They may not even be marketable and so cannot be included in the measures of national accounts.

We do not go so far as to say that the human capital approach ought never to be used. However, it should always be accompanied by explicit acknowledgment of its shortcomings and used only if the client for the analysis insists upon it after having considered the alternatives.

The decision-maker approach—the safe passage?

Having successfully negotiated a passage around both Scylla and Charybdis, we now turn to our suggested way forward. It may have become clear by now that underlying the discussion so far is a centrally recurring issue that relates to objectives, i.e., what are we trying to accomplish, and on whose authority? Addressing this question occupies the rest of this chapter.

Implicit in the perfect market approach is the maximand of the total sum of expected utilities. Implicit in the human capital approach is the maximand of national income, Gross Domestic Product or Gross National Product. Implicit in many ergonomic studies is the maximand of worker safety. In others, the criteria are narrowly commercial and the implicit maximand is profit. Implicit in many health care evaluations is the maximand of health. A related set of issues concerns matters of equity. How is fairness or social justice defined, on whose authority, and how ought they to be embodied in economic evaluations? Addressing each of these issues requires the exercise of judgment and, in particular, that critically important subset of judgments generally known as social value judgments. We turn to these now.

Making the unavoidable value judgments explicitly

There are at least three broad approaches that a reasonable person might adopt in addressing the value judgments embedded in methods of evaluating workplace interventions. The first is to adopt an ethical convention commonly employed in a particular discipline, conventions such as 'workplace safety' or 'utility maximization'. Two advantages to such a choice are that it has probably been thoroughly worked over and understood, and that one can communicate with fellow disciplinarians on the basis of an immediately shared understanding of concepts, theories, and their applications. However, this approach has little intrinsic ethical merit, and some downsides are that the convention's weaknesses may have been glossed over or largely ignored. Thus, maximizing workplace safety carries the baggage that it suggests every reduction in workplace hazards is worth undertaking. Utility maximization carries the baggage that it is only individual welfares of a particular kind that matter. Moreover, although communication with fellow disciplinarians may be facilitated, communication with fellow transdisciplinarians may be difficult.

The second approach is to seek to discover what society thinks are the appropriate value judgments to make. In pursuing this line, one might trawl public utterances by those with public responsibility, such as departmental ministers, to discover whether labour market, health, or employment policy is about maximizing utility, national income, health, or something else. This is not an easy task, but if accomplished will give an analysis the moral authority that the previous approach lacked, as well as a direct communications bridge of understanding. The main reasons why this is not an easy task is that public utterances of the required sort are few in number, nearly always ambiguous, at an unsuitably high level of generality, and often contradictory. Moreover, there are major empirical problems of construct validity and measurement that remain. There is a further problem: the list of possible maximands rises as one trawls ministries. This gives rise to three questions. First, is it sensible somehow to combine the plurality of objectives in an overall social welfare function? Secondly, how are the trade-offs between them to be made? Thirdly, what ought the analyst do about any omitted plausible aims and objectives that no one claims for their own?

The third approach is to create a professional scientific consensus, a kind of reference case (Gold *et al.* 1996), that permits all potential perspectives, objectives and trade-offs to be taken into account, and that for any particular study design enables the scope of the analysis, including its perspective, to be selected according to the values and intentions of the stakeholders on whose behalf the study is done. The consensus group we have in mind is the multi-disciplinary and multi-professional group of researchers who investigate the merits of OHS interventions.

This third approach might involve guessing at what the public utterances would be if they were made less ambiguously and without contradiction, and adopting them as one's ethical basis. Alternatively, it might involve seeking a consensus from the ranks of fellow scientists or seeking a consensus from amongst those deemed to be stakeholders. It might be eclectic, seeking to approach evaluative questions in a flexible way, depending on who were the main clients for the research, or in multiple ways by evaluating workplace interventions from more than one perspective, thus exposing important possible differences in the values of different stakeholders.

We think it is worth trying to build a professional scientific consensus based on a reasoned attempt to distil what government, workers, workers' families, employers, workers' compensation boards, health and safety regulators, and other third party payers, indeed, any stakeholder is seeking to achieve. It can be changed as the distilling becomes more refined or as the things distilled themselves change with the changing political scene. It would be desirable to adopt practical tools derived from it that are used elsewhere in the same jurisdiction. This may be the best way forward on the grounds that, done well, the professional approach may come to be seen as 'the approach': the one most persuasive on ethical grounds and, with time, the one most acceptable through familiarity and clear understanding.

A pragmatist objects

In the health and safety literature there is a robust tradition of pragmatism, so one may readily anticipate a pragmatic objection. It runs along the following lines: theoretical discussion of means and ends, efficiency and equity, science and ethics, social welfare, and the like are rather beside the point. The real point is that decisions on health and safety are taken on the basis of their impact on the bottom line. Do they enhance productivity and, if so, do they do so sufficiently to warrant their undoubted cost to employers? That is all there is to it. The only question for the analyst is to measure the bottom line effect. There can be little doubt that this has been the focus of much of the evaluative literature on workplace health and safety interventions in the past. More recently, researchers have begun to pay attention to the measurement of health effects—but still largely for instrumental reasons; that is, that they generate beneficial productivity and, hence, bottom line consequences. The hope, of course, is that business managers will be more likely to listen to health and safety staff, who are all too often at the margins of operational decision making and become allies in the diffusion of interventions for safety throughout the business.

This is a powerful argument. Even though it makes fairly heroic assumptions about what it is that motivates management, it is an argument that scientists ignore at their peril. The pragmatist is, however, only half right. The bottom line does, indeed, matter and the impact of interventions on it needs to be evaluated, but the employers' bottom line is not the only such line and it would seem wise to consider the balance of advantage over disadvantage from all relevant points of view. Moreover, in order to know whether the intervention is one worth supporting in the first place, a broader evaluative framework is implied that takes everyone's interests into account, including the distributional and redistributional consequences.

Two critical levels of analysis

We propose that there are two critical levels at which evaluative research must operate. One level addresses the question 'ought this intervention to be adopted?' The second level addresses the question 'what is the best way of encouraging the intervention in question to be adopted?'

The first question seeks to discover what ought to be done. The natural perspective from which to consider this question entails a social value judgment that we suggest be as uncontroversial as possible. Therefore, we propose that the perspective from which this question is addressed be explicit and universal. Our suggestion is for the perspective also to be the societal one; that is, inclusive of the health and safety consequences for all possible stakeholders. The advantages of this approach are several. First, it becomes clear which benefits and costs, and to whom, are to be included, so that any bias arising out of a less than comprehensive inventory is exposed and minimized. Second, its starting point is one in which any cost or benefit can, in principle, be included in the analysis, making the informational content as complete as possible. Third, for practical purposes, it enumerates an agenda of costs and benefits that can be further considered by the decision-making clients for inclusion or exclusion according to their, rather than the analyst's, values. Fourth, it enables a comprehensive view of distributional and redistributional effects to be taken into account, so that they can be traced, assessed, and their acceptability addressed. Distributional effects are usually important factors in determining the social desirability of interventions. This inclusive and universal perspective was also that proposed by the Washington Panel (Gold *et al.* 1996).

The second question addresses issues of whose interest it is, or is not, for the intervention to be adopted, what instruments might be needed in order to persuade those whose interests it does not match voluntarily to adopt it, or what instruments of regulation and control might be used that force them involuntarily to adopt it. In most cases, the benefits and costs of greater health and safety will not be distributed equally across all stakeholder groups. This asymmetry should not to be ignored by analysts, and empirical research that seeks to assess the significance of such costs and benefits, whether quantitatively or qualitatively, seems to be the best way to work out what type of encouragement (e.g., a subsidy or some form of cost sharing) might be effective in gaining consent in circumstances where the workplace decision makers are not convinced of the dominance of advantage over disadvantage from their own perspective. It seems also to be wise for researchers to establish the likely size and location of any political resistance that would arise to regulatory solutions. Here, the emphasis is not on the inherent fairness or unfairness of the consequences of an intervention, but on its acceptability to all affected parties, in order to focus on the policy implementation issues of persuasion, compensation and enforcement.

A specific proposal and some of its implications

We seek to define a value-laden end which can serve as the basis for evaluating OHS interventions, one that is relatively immune to the criticisms of the perfect market approach, one that does not treat people as carthorses, but is infused with a clear humanity, one that will enable comparisons to be made across similar activities within the jurisdiction, such as health care and road safety, so as to avoid significantly different investment criteria being used, one that preferably uses or adapts instruments that are widely available and whose characteristics are well-understood, one that will enable matters of fairness and distributive equity to be addressed explicitly and analytically, and one that addresses the informational needs both of workplace parties and of the wider community.

To this end, we propose three broad framework principles for evaluative analyses. The first ethical proposition is:

- *The prime objective of health and safety interventions is to enhance the expected health-related welfare of individuals in the workplace. It is not to enhance expected utility or national income.*

Supplementary objectives might include health-related welfare effects on others, such as family members and care-givers, effects described earlier as externalities. The perspective from which such evaluations ought to take place is thus narrower than the societal one advocated by many economists (e.g., Gold *et al.* 1996), but it is different from and broader than the narrow focus on the business bottom line. It will be necessary to determine the scope of cost effects that one routinely ought to take account of, as in a reference case (Gold *et al.* 1996). This step also involves making social value judgments. There is a strong case to be made for flexibility in the choice of perspective, since studies may reasonably take different views on the grounds that responsibility for managing resources varies from one situation to another. Common to all evaluations is a focus on those working in the workplaces and likely to participate in, benefit from or incur costs as a result of the interventions. Where the emphasis should lie in any particular study will be a matter for prior determination by researchers working with research commissioners. The second ethical proposition is:

- *The perspective of particular evaluative studies will be determined in conjunction with relevant stakeholders and supplemented where necessary by analyses that incorporate significant external effects.*

The purpose here is to enable a clear focus both on the pragmatist's concern, such as the bottom line, and the wider interests of other stakeholders. To take an extreme example, a costly workplace intervention whose benefit falls entirely on workers and their families in the form of health, and which has no productivity impact, may be amply justified in social terms, but may not be in any individual employer's interest to implement.

The third ethical proposition concerns equity:

- *Economic evaluations should, in addition to considering efficiency, identify potential equity issues of significance in conjunction with stakeholders and always present results in a way that reveals how the incidence of costs and benefits falls both immediately and after any predictable market adjustments have been made.*

The distribution of costs and benefits is important not only so that matters of equity can be addressed, but also in order to facilitate thinking about how an intervention might best be implemented. Identifying the incidence of costs and benefits is more difficult than may appear at first to non-economists in that changing costs of production will usually generate consequential changes in the type and amount of resources that businesses will employ, with further consequences for prices and wages (see Box 2.5 for definitions). Thus, a cost that may initially appear to be borne by employers might, as time goes by, come to be passed on to consumers in the form of higher prices and/or to workers in the form of lower wages. Such effects will have implications not only for the assessment of the desirability of an intervention, but also for that of its implementation. For example, there seems little point in compensating employers for cost-increasing measures if the negative consequences for employers have been passed on to the consumers in the form of higher prices of their products.

What is a little more health and safety worth?

A little more health and safety is not of infinite value. If it were, economic evaluation of workplace interventions to enhance health and safety would be unnecessary. The need for evaluation arises because the benefits are not infinite, because they are uncertain, because they come with a price tag, and because each of these has an impact that is different from one stakeholder group to another.

Box 2.5 The meaning of incidence

Incidence in epidemiology: the number of new cases of a health condition occurring in a population during a period of time (compared with *prevalence*, which is the number of cases of a health condition in a given population at a specific date).

Incidence in economics: the entities that bear the cost of an intervention or receive its benefit (compare *initial incidence*, which is the apparent or legal impact, with *final incidence*, which is the impact after all consequential adjustments have occurred).

There can be a considerable difference between the two kinds of economic incidence, initial incidence and final incidence. For example, employers might be taxed, whether for OHS or other purpose, but the tax may be effectively shifted to employees and/or consumers. The extent to which this happens depends on the motivation of the firm and the characteristics of demand and supply.

Taking a broad view across an economy, it seems highly likely that the relationship between the size of benefit and the number of interventions will be non-linear. A stylized example is portrayed in Figure 2.2. In this example we assume that interventions are ranked from left to right in descending order of their additional contribution to the benefit. Thus, on the far left, machine guards are fitted to those machines most likely to cause serious injury. As one moves rightward, there lie guards applied to machines that are less likely to cause a hazardous event and/or have events that are less damaging. On the far right are guards applied to machines that pose virtually no threat to health and safety at all. The cumulative benefit always rises as the number of interventions increases, although it does so at a diminishing rate. At any one time an economy may be located at particular points on this curve such as *a* or *b*, where *b* represents an economy that has invested more in health and safety than the economy at *a*. A more realistic picture might be that different sectors of an economy are at different points. So, if we suppose that the manufacturing and the transport sectors each face the same functional relationship shown in the figure, one sector may be at point *a* and the other at point *b*.

Even if we had sufficient information to form a judgment about the shape and height of the curve in Figure 2.2, this would be insufficient to determine where on the curve one ought to locate. The flat of the curve is an unlikely segment to choose, but there is plainly much scope for choice in the region

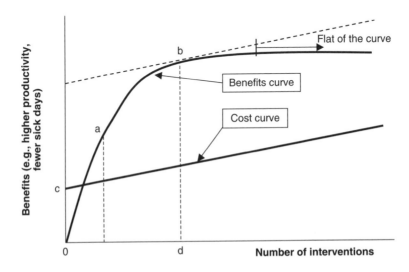

Fig. 2.2 Conceptualization of the relationship between interventions and consequences.

to its left. The missing information is the costs of the interventions, which we may assume not to fall as interventions increase. Making the simplifying assumption that these rise at a constant rate from c, the optimal location is determined at point d. Additional interventions beyond that point cost more than the amount of benefit they bring. At points to the left of d additional interventions add more benefit than they cost. At this point the slopes of the two curves are equal—marginal cost equals marginal benefit.

Despite its high degree of simplification, Figure 2.2 represents the essential character of the solution to the question 'what is a little more health and safety worth?' The answer depends on a balancing of cost and benefits, disadvantage and advantage, with a presumption that those projects whose benefits exceed costs ought to be adopted and those for which that is not true ought not.

The rest of the book will develop this fundamental model and extend it in various ways, for example, by considering the distribution of consequences in the evaluation, taking account of risk and uncertainty, the duration of costs and benefits, and exploring in greater detail the characteristics that make for high quality research studies of workplace interventions.

Chapter 3

A critical review of the application of economic evaluation methodologies in occupational health and safety

Emile Tompa, Roman Dolinschi,
Karen Niven, and Claire de Oliveira

Introduction

With limited time and competing demands on scarce funds, many organizations are apt to focus only on those occupational health and safety (OHS) issues that are required by law, or the ones demonstrated to have an impact on the bottom line. Prevention initiatives may not always bring financial returns, yet if an intervention has health and safety benefits, then it still may be a good business decision for some organizations. Essentially, doing a good job of health and safety is regarded by some organizations as a critical part of business, and is considered a key benefit in its own right. Nonetheless, information on the costs and consequences of an OHS intervention is an invaluable input into the decision of whether or not to undertake it.

After embarking on a systematic literature review of OHS interventions with economic analyses (Tompa *et al.* 2007a) we discovered that few intervention studies undertook such analyses. Of those that did, the quality of analyses was generally low. Other reviews of the OHS literature have similar findings (Goossens *et al.* 1999; Niven 2002; DeRango and Franzini 2003). Indeed, a common complaint in the assessments of the research literature on the economic evaluation of workplace interventions is that 'well-designed and conducted evaluations of programme costs and benefits were nearly impossible to find' (Niven 2002).

Many studies that undertake economic analyses focus exclusively on workers' compensation costs. Yet, changes in workers' compensation costs are a poor proxy of the health and other resource implications of an intervention introduced to avert occupational injury and disease. Indirect costs, such as recruitment and training costs incurred for replacing injured workers, costs associated with accommodating injured worker, and lost home production are all costs not normally captured by workers' compensation. These, too, are not a complete list of costs borne by organizations, workers, and society. Examples of other costs include home care provided by family members and the direct value of health lost by an individual. Moreover, only a fraction of occupational injuries and diseases are formally reported to worker compens-ation authorities (Shannon and Lowe 2002).

Essentially, a broad perspective is needed to capture a fuller range of costs associated with occupational injuries and diseases, and the resource implications of efforts to avert them. With a narrow perspective, an intervention that shifts costs to another stakeholder may appear as a value added to some, even if the net benefit across all stakeholders is negative. Knowledge of the full range of costs and consequences and their distribution across stakeholders can help identify interventions for which public support is warranted due to their health and other benefits, but which are unlikely to be supported independently by the private sector due to the uneven distribution of costs and consequences (see Chapter 2 for a fuller treatment of this issue).

One reason few intervention studies undertake an economic evaluation is due to the lack of appropriate competencies among OHS researchers, since their expertise tends to focus on the evaluation of health effectiveness, rather than cost-effective. Undertaking an economic evaluation requires the expertise of someone with training in these methods, and we highly recommend that a researcher with such a background be part of the evaluation team from the outset (see Chapter 7 for further discussion of this issue).

Undertaking economic evaluations of OHS interventions can be difficult for a number of reasons. Most economic evaluation methods texts in the health care field give little guidance on how best to confront these difficulties, since most are designed for use in clinical settings and are difficult to adapt to workplace contexts. Following are some of the challenges confronted in the OHS arena:

- the policy arena of OHS and labour legislation is complex, with multiple stakeholders and sometimes conflicting incentives and priorities;
- there are substantial differences in the perceptions of health risks associated with work experiences amongst workplace parties and policymakers;
- the burden of costs and consequences may be borne by different stakeholders in the system;
- there are multiple providers of indemnity and medical care coverage, and no one measure captures the full cost of occupational injury and disease;

- industry-specific human resources practices (e.g., hiring temporary workers, self-employed contract, farming out non-core activities) can make it difficult to identify all occupational injuries and diseases;
- the dearth of data available from organizations on costs and consequences can make it challenging and expensive to obtain good measures.

In many cases the distinction is blurred between developing a business case for health and safety, and undertaking a full-fledged economic evaluation of an OHS intervention. The two serve different purposes and, although the methodologies have some common ground, there can be substantial differences between them. A business case generally refers to analyses designed specifically to support organizational decision making. Comprehensive quantitative analyses of costs and consequences are not always necessary to provide evidence for decision making, since managers often make decisions based on a combination of tangible and intangible benefits (Marsden *et al.* 2004). A business case generally takes the perspective of the firm, but it does not necessarily focus exclusively on identifying positive financial returns. Factors of interest in a business case can include 'getting health and safety right', improving productivity, avoiding certain costs, meeting client demands, and improving staff morale (Marsden *et al.* 2004).

An economic evaluation can also present the business case, but generally goes much further. It is customary to consider a more comprehensive list of costs and consequences accruing to various stakeholders in the OHS arena and to those outside it, such as workers, employers, insurers, health care providers, family members of workers, and society at large. It is also customary to undertake sensitivity analysis of key elements of uncertainty in order to test the robustness of results. Other qualities include a fuller reporting of context, formulation of measures, and computational underpinnings of analyses in order to allow for a better sense of generalizability and transferability than a business case might generally present.

In this chapter we draw from an environmental scan and systematic review of OHS intervention studies with economic analyses undertaken by the authors (Tompa *et al.* 2006, 2007a) to identify the key areas where improvements could be made in the application of these methodologies.

Methodological issues identified

In reviewing OHS intervention studies with economic analyses, we grouped methodological shortcomings into ten issues, which we categorized under three groups: study design and related factors, measurement and analytic factors, and computational and reporting factors.

The intent in highlighting these methodological issues is to provide insight into how to take the application of economic evaluation methodology further in future studies. In what follows we elaborate on each of the ten issues.

Study design and related factors

Issue 1: study design

Study design is closely tied to the evaluation of the effectiveness of an intervention, but it also bears on the economic evaluation, particularly with regard to means of capturing the magnitude of consequences. The merits of different epidemiological designs are well documented (see Chapter 8 in this text, as well as Lilienfeld and Stolley 1994; Rothman and Greenland 1998). Most workplace intervention researchers would argue that randomized controlled trials are the design of choice, but non-randomized controlled studies, interrupted time series, and simple before-and-after studies can also be well executed and provide valuable information. Many of the intervention studies we identified that had economic analyses were based on before-and-after study design without randomization or concurrent controls (see, for example, Tadano 1990; Thompson 1990; Bradley 1996; Baxter and Harrison 2000; Lewis *et al.* 2002).

The main failing we found with many studies was the attribution of all changes in the outcome of interest to the intervention, without accounting for confounding factors. In all study designs, but particularly with before-and-after designs, known or conjectured confounders that are not controlled for through randomization ought to be controlled for in some other way, for example, through multivariate modelling techniques using interrupted time series data. This is the approach taken by Lanoie and Tavenas (1996); the researchers controlled for several individual demographic, employment, and other contextual characteristics through regression modelling in order to assess the effectiveness of a participatory ergonomics intervention in reducing occupational back injuries amongst workers at a warehouse distribution centre. With some interventions, individual micro-data may not be available, but similar techniques can also be used with departmental, plant, or firm-level data.

Many macro-level factors merit careful consideration, but are often ignored in intervention studies. In particular, the declining injury rates observed in jurisdictions in North America and other locations over the last decade or so may be an important factor to consider in the analysis, since the trend-level improvement in the outcome measure of interest can be easily, yet inappropriately, attributed to the intervention under consideration. Baxter and Harrison (2000), for example, showed a downward trend in the percentage of operators reporting musculoskeletal injuries over a seven-year period, four years of which were prior to the intervention, but nonetheless failed to adjust for the impact of this downward trend on the outcome of interest.

Randomization is preferred, but often not possible. Even with randomization and concurrent controls, there may still be pre-existing, pre-intervention differences that bear on the outcomes of interest. Controlling for pre-existing conditions and other confounders can be undertaken through regression modelling techniques. This was the approach taken by DeRango *et al.* (2003), even though the subjects were partly randomized to control and intervention arms, and concurrent controls were used. Specifically, the researchers took a three-step approach to ensure that they had correctly identified the effects of the intervention on the outcome: first, they had partial randomization of subjects between the two intervention groups and a control group, since full randomization was not feasible due to the possibility of knowledge sharing between groups; second, they employed a quasi-experimental study design using a concurrent control group; and third, they used regression modelling to assess the consequences side of the intervention, controlling for a variety of contextual factors. In addition, the study design specified data collection requirements for dependent and independent variables prior to the implementation of the two interventions in order to control for any pre-existing differences between treatment and control groups at baseline that may predict health and productivity.

Issue 2: study perspective

Most economic evaluations of workplace interventions we identified were conducted from the perspective of the firm. Some exceptions are Arnetz *et al.* (2003), Greenwood *et al.* (1990), and Loisel *et al.* (2002), which took the perspective of a workers' compensation insurance provider, and Jensen *et al.* (2001), which took a societal perspective. In many studies the perspective was not explicitly stated, but simply implied to be that of the company and, in fact, we noted in some studies an inconsistent treatment of costs and consequences relative to their implied perspective (details are described in 'Issue 5: valuation of costs and consequences'). In some cases, researchers may present their analyses from a company perspective, but are really seeking to persuade the company of the merits of an intervention that serves the workers' point of view.

There is a strong normative argument for considering a broad, societal perspective, and for considering the distribution of costs and consequences across various stakeholders (see Chapter 2 for a thorough discussion of this recommendation). Specifically, the fact that there are multiple stakeholders affected by OHS issues (firms, workers and their families, unions, health care providers, insurers, society) suggests that costs and consequences borne by all the stakeholders ought to be included in the analysis. This is the norm in other economic evaluation contexts where there are multiple stakeholders (e.g., environmental impact assessment). A broad perspective does not preclude providing information on other perspectives. In fact, a disaggregation of costs and consequences would be invaluable, as it would provide insight into their distribution.

Issue 3: measurement time frame and sustainability

The purpose of most, if not all, OHS interventions is to have a long-lasting impact on the OHS performance of a firm. Yet, few studies have the luxury of a measurement time frame long enough to assess sustainability of the intervention effects. The concern here is that the observed change in OHS indicators due to the intervention (even if properly measured and attributed) may be a one-time, short-lived effect, rather than a long-lasting and sustainable change. A related issue is that OHS performance can vary dramatically from year to year in ways that are unrelated to the intervention, and a longer measurement time frame in conjunction with the use of regression modelling techniques might help separate the noise from the true impact. Some studies also noted a Hawthorne effect, in which the training component of an intervention increased both awareness and reporting of injuries.

In some studies the time frame was not sufficient to observe a measurable and statistically significant impact of the intervention. This can particularly be an issue with long-onset conditions, such as some musculoskeletal injuries. In such cases, the full magnitude of health impacts can be assessed via intermediate outcomes that can be influenced by the intervention in the short run and that are empirically linked to final outcomes. Clearly, some knowledge of the epidemiology of disease or injury is required to correctly determine the minimum necessary length of measurement time frame. Accounting for future consequences that extend beyond the measurement time period might also be considered. Few studies extrapolated costs and consequences into the future (for an exception, see Lanoie and Tavenas 1996). If one takes this approach, assumptions underlying the projections should be well grounded, and their impact on the results should be tested through sensitivity analysis. Extrapolation is a highly debated issue, which we discuss under 'Issue 6: analytical time frame and future consequences'.

Measurement and analytic factors

Issue 4: consideration of all important costs and consequences

The majority of studies that did undertake some form of economic analysis considered only consequences in monetary terms, but did not consider intervention costs. These are not full economic evaluations since they stop one step short of a full evaluation.

Amongst the studies that undertook a full economic evaluation, many considered only a subset of costs and consequences. For example, in an evaluation of a workstation redesign and education program, Bradley (1996) measured the costs of engineering evaluation and workstation redesign, but not employee time for training. In an office ergonomics intervention, Richardson (2002) considered the cost of an ergonomics assessment and purchase of new equipment, but not the costs of time devoted to installation and training. Similarly, in an evaluation of an ergonomic workstation redesign and training program, Tadano (1990) included the costs of therapist time, but not the costs of workstation redesign, training, or time for mini-breaks. Two studies that are more thorough in their consideration of costs and consequences are Lanoie and Tavenas (1996), and Loisel et al. (2002).

Most studies that undertook economic analyses focused on workers' compensation claim costs and medical care costs (e.g., Tadano 1990; Bradley 1996; Baxter and Harrison 2000; Lewis et al. 2002; Richardson 2002). However, using workers' compensation claims as the sole or primary health outcome may fall short of providing an accurate or complete picture of the health benefits of an intervention. Many compensable injuries and diseases go unreported (Shannon and Lowe 2002), and others are not compensable. A related issue is that workers' compensation benefits are simply transfers and do not reflect the full set of costs and consequences borne by different stakeholders (a more detailed discussion of transfers can be found in 'Issue 5: valuation of costs and consequences', and the topic is given full treatment in Chapter 10). Researchers might consider other measures of health and their associated costs, either through primary data collection or use of other administrative data sources (e.g., first aid reports, records of modified duty, private indemnity claims, and short-term absenteeism).

Though some studies considered proxies for productivity such as absenteeism, only a few considered explicit measures of productivity or product and service quality. Identifying measures of productivity can be a challenge; though some studies were quite creative in exploiting administrative data sources within the firm (see, for example, Nerhood and Rael 1995; DeRango et al. 2003; see also Chapter 7 for strategies to deal with data dearth issues).

Issue 5: valuation of costs and consequences

Accurate valuation of costs and consequences can present critical challenges that are not apparent at first blush. Three items in particular stand out: identifying prices that correctly reflect the value of resources embodied in the costs and consequences under consideration, identifying prices that are consistent with the perspective taken, and measuring incremental costs and consequences attributable to an intervention, rather than the total costs incurred and consequences realized (valuation issues are given full treatment in Chapters 10 and 11).

Regarding the first item, prices should be based on the true worth of a good or service, i.e., the opportunity or resource costs embodied in it (see Chapter 4 for a fuller treatment of this issue). If a well-functioning market exists for a good or service, then the 'sticker price' (nominal market price) will accurately reflect this worth. In some cases a well-functioning market does not exist and, therefore, the 'sticker price' may not be a good measure or may not be available. In such cases, economists attempt to estimate a 'shadow price' to better reflect the opportunity or resource cost. A good example of this issue is presented in a study by DeRango et al. (2003). The study is of a new, highly adjustable chair introduced to a state governmental agency that collects sales taxes. The incremental taxes collected by workers who were provided a new chair and training were estimated to be $US 25,398 per worker per year. However, taxes are simply transfers, and transfers often net out to zero at the societal level. In the DeRango et al. (2003) study, the shadow price of the incremental increase in productivity of the tax collectors attributable to the intervention is likely much lower than the incremental taxes collected by them. At one level the question is whether a dollar in the public sector is worth more than a dollar in the private sector to society, given the current distribution of resources between the two sectors. It may be that the current distribution is deemed optimal, in which case incremental transfers to the government have no value at the societal level. An alternative approach would be to consider the level of employment at the tax collecting agency that would be sufficient to maintain the optimal level of taxation. An intervention that maintains this optimal level with lower level of labour input would be considered a valued productivity improvement. The investigators of the chair study used as an alternative value the percentage of increased taxes collected multiplied by the wage rate (based on the notion that the wage rate reflects the marginal product of a worker).

Thompson (1990) also used transfers to value consequences. Specifically, the researcher undertook an evaluation of a paid exercise break program designed to reduce musculoskeletal strain in the data-entry office of a large California public utility. One of the functions performed by the data-entry staff was processing customer cheques. The more expedient processing of cheques resulted in substantial increases in interest earned by the utility ($US 130,992 per annum) due to earlier withdrawal of funds from customer accounts. Once again, for reasons stated earlier, this measure may not reflect the true value of the productivity consequences of the exercise program.

The concern of inaccurate valuation might also arise when prices are generated within a firm for accounting purposes to allow for transfers and billing between departments. If these prices do not reflect true market prices, one can look to the market to identify costs for similar products or services. In some cases market prices can also be inappropriate when a competitive market does not exist, and an extra premium is paid for a good or service (e.g., specialty clinician services, new pharmaceutical products). In this case, adjustment needs to be made to the market price, possibly by turning to comparable products and services.

The second key item, identifying prices that are consistent with the perspective taken, can arise when several stakeholders share costs or consequences. This is particularly relevant for insurance expenses covered by third-party payers, e.g., workers' compensation, medical care, and private indemnity insurance. Since many firms are not fully experience rated, the full cost of a claim will not be billed to the firm. As noted, workers' compensation cost savings were one of the most frequently considered consequences in the studies we identified, yet few studies conducted from the perspective of the firm adjusted the wage replacement and health care costs borne by the insurer to reflect the fraction of these costs that would be billed back to the company in the form of higher premiums. One exception is Lanoie and Tavenas (1996). In this study the researchers consulted the firm's financial analyst for an estimate of the costs to the firm of a day of workers' compensation paid absence. If a societal perspective is taken, then the cost to an insurer will underestimate the true costs, since workers often share in the burden through co-payments (i.e., benefits that are less than their lost wages), and both the worker and the employer incur expenses that are not covered by an insurer.

The third key item is the need to consider incremental (marginal) consequences and costs attributable to an intervention, rather than the total consequences and costs. At issue is the fact that some of the costs incurred during the intervention period would be incurred even if the status quo or comparator option were chosen. Similarly, certain health consequences realized during or after the intervention would have been realized even without the intervention (due to other factors), so assessing the total health effects observed in relation to the intervention would be inaccurate. Since two or more programmes are being compared in an economic evaluation, one is interested in identifying the incremental costs and consequences attributable to the intervention in question. For example, the total cost of the purchase of a workstation and related equipment may not be fully attributable to an ergonomics intervention if a similar purchase was already planned. Only the incremental cost of purchasing a more expensive, ergonomically enhanced workstation and equipment would be relevant. Most studies we identified attributed the total costs incurred during the intervention period to the intervention under investigation, although in a few studies researchers made the effort to identify the incremental costs. For example, in Lanoie and Tavenas (1996) the researchers consulted the company's equipment replacement policy to identify the incremental costs of equipment associated with the participatory ergonomics programme. In Loisel *et al.* (2002) the researchers made efforts to distinguish between standard expenses incurred by the insurer for treatment of back injuries from incremental expenses attributable to the particular back pain management intervention under study.

Issue 6: analytical time frame and future costs and consequences

In many cases, substantial costs and consequences may occur after the measurement time period. The projection of costs and consequences beyond the period of measurement is a highly debated issue (Drummond and Sculpher 2005) and the validity of such projections rests on the quality of the data that they are drawn from. Clearly, there is a risk of overstating the benefits, particularly if there is the possibility of decreased effectiveness of the intervention over time. In such cases, a sensitivity analysis should be undertaken to assess the robustness of projections to the assumptions underlying them. Most of the studies we identified took the conservative 'stop-and-drop' approach in which no costs or consequences are assumed after the measurement time period, but did not comment on the probable bias this introduced. One study, Lanoie and Tavenas (1996), considered both the stop-and-drop scenario and a scenario in which consequences are realized for five years into the future. The researchers found that the participatory ergonomics intervention evaluated in the study was financially rewarding for the firm only in the second scenario. They did not test their extrapolation assumptions by considering different scenarios for the future, though a sensitivity analysis was performed on the discount rate.

Issue 7: adjustment for inflation and time preference

Adjustment for time preference through discounting is critical if the costs and/or consequences of an intervention are realized over more than one year. If prices are expressed in nominal dollars from different calendar years, one should also adjust for inflation. It is generally advisable to first make adjustments for inflation, and then discount the costs and consequences expressed in constant dollars (or another monetary metric) to a base year. Discounting is required for both costs and consequences, even if consequences are not measured in monetary terms. Many jurisdictions stipulate the discount rate at which public sector investments are to be discounted. For the private sector, firms may have their own specific rate used for project investments. The real discount rate recommended by several researchers for discounting constant dollars to a particular calendar year is 3% (Gold *et al.* 1996; Goossens *et al.* 1999; Haddix *et al.* 2003), but because a number of studies in the past used 5%, it is recommended to consider both rates in an analysis. Undertaking a sensitivity analysis using a range of rates from 0 to 10% is also recommended (Haddix *et al.* 2003). In general, it is recommended to use the real discount rate, and not the nominal rate that includes both the time value of money and the rate of inflation. Separating inflation from the time preference component allows one to address any variation or uncertainty about inflation separately without confusing it with the time value of money. Also, varying the discount rate alone to test the robustness of results is not adequate sensitivity analysis in most cases, although it is the most common and sometimes the only kind of sensitivity analysis undertaken. There are many other aspects of uncertainty beyond the discount rate that need to be addressed in order to test the robustness of results. A sensitivity analysis should also present the reasons for the specific estimates employed.

Many of the studies we identified did not appear to adjust for inflation or time preference before aggregating monies from different time periods. For example, in Bradley (1996) the researcher described an ergonomics program introduced to address cumulative trauma disorders (CTD) in an office environment that was evaluated over several years. Prior to the programme (1991–1992), health care costs for five cases of CTD totalled $US 63,628.98 (or $US 12,725.80 per case), whereas after the introduction of the programme there were 35 cases over the 1993–1994 period with costs of health care, engineering evaluation, and changes to workstations totalling $US 2,886.25 (or $US 82.46 per case). The researcher made no mention of adjusting health care or other costs for inflation, or discounting costs to a particular calendar year. A good example of adjusting for inflation and time preference is a study of a participatory ergonomics programme in a warehouse distribution centre by Lanoie and Tavenas (1996). Direct and indirect costs from 1991 to 1998 were discounted to the 1989 calendar year with a nominal discount rate of 11.5% that incorporated both inflation and time preference. Analysis of the sensitivity of results to the discount factor was tested by recalculating the net present value using 5, 10, and 15% rates.

Issue 8: use of assumptions and treatment of uncertainty

Resource allocation decisions are invariably conducted in the context of uncertainty and incomplete information. Both need to be addressed in any analytical methods. A distinction is generally made between statistical uncertainty and uncertainty related to other aspects of the intervention. For the former, confidence intervals are used to describe the range in which the true value may lie. The latter is often associated with incomplete information on the costs and consequences of the intervention. This may necessitate the use of proxy measures, information from alternative data sources, and invariably, the use of assumptions. Assumptions need to be well grounded and justified. Sensitivity analysis is usually undertaken to test the robustness of results to variations in key assumptions. There are various approaches to conducting sensitivity analysis across multiple dimensions [e.g., multi-way sensitivity analysis, threshold analysis, scenario analysis, probabilistic sensitivity analysis (see Chapter 12; see also Claxton *et al.* 2005; Drummond and Sculpher 2005)].

The above principles were not always followed in the studies we identified. For example, Bradley (1996) concluded that the intervention was effective on the basis of the reduction in the severity (not incidence) of cumulative trauma disorders (CTDs) after the introduction of the intervention. The number of CTDs post-intervention, however, had actually increased seven-fold (from 5 to 35 CTDs). The inherent assumption was that the 35 CTDs would have occurred without the intervention and each of them would have been as severe as the five pre-intervention CTDs, if not for the intervention. Once again, no sensitivity analysis was undertaken. Lanoie and Tavenas (1996) estimated the number of prevented occupational back injuries to be 6, 11, and 15 during the three years of the active intervention phase based on regression modelling results. In extrapolating into the future, the researchers assumed that the number of prevented back injuries from the last year forward would remain at 15 a year. The positive net present value identified from the ten-year analytic time frame appears highly contingent upon this assumption, yet no sensitivity analysis was undertaken around it. Finally, few of the studies we reviewed addressed the statistical uncertainty of the study results.

Computational and reporting factors

Issue 9: choice of summary measure

Choosing between one of the three key types of economic evaluation [cost–benefit analysis (CBA), cost-effectiveness analysis (CEA), and cost–utility analysis (CUA)] should be based on the objective of the intervention and the question being addressed by the study. These, in turn, are influenced by the nature of the key outcome variable and the perspective being taken. For example, if the perspective is that of a private sector firm, CBA might be preferred if the key objective of an intervention is to reduce workers' compensation premiums through improved OHS performance. The three types of evaluation differ primarily in the measurement of the outcome (monetary metric for CBA, natural units for CEA, and utility metric for CUA), and each has its strengths and weaknesses (see Chapter 9; Drummond *et al.* 2005; Haddix *et al.* 2003 for details).

CBA is by no means a gold standard for economic evaluation of health and safety interventions, since it can fail to account adequately for many aspects of the health consequences realized by an intervention. A number of issues arise when placing a monetary value on health and life (see Chapters 2 and 5; DeRango and Franzini 2003; Haddix *et al.* 2003; Drummond *et al.* 2005 for details), and there is merit in considering more than one type of analysis in any particular study in order to provide insight into the outcomes of interest. For example, one could undertake a CEA to better capture the health outcomes that are not readily translatable into a monetary metric (e.g., pain reduction, MSK disorders averted), and a CBA in which health outcomes are evaluated by allotting a monetary measure (e.g., willingness to pay, reduced productivity, cost of absences). This is the approach taken by Loisel *et al.* (2002) in their study (i.e., they undertook both CEA and CBA). Most of the studies we identified with a full evaluation undertook a CBA, which is consistent with the literature on workplace-based interventions. A few studies undertook a CEA, and no studies undertook a CUA.

Issue 10: reporting issues

For a study to be useful to decision makers, it must provide new and relevant information. Transferability of an intervention to other settings requires sufficient information to assess its applicability or generalizability. Information that assists with this process includes details about the context, nature of the intervention, timing, magnitude, and the type, amount, and variability of costs and consequences. At another level, clear and complete reporting facilitates the reader's ability to assess the quality of a study, or simply understand what assumptions and calculations were made to arrive at a final value.

In several of the studies we reviewed, the reporting of context, measures, computational formulas, and assumptions was modest, making it difficult to determine how values were derived, evaluate the quality of the analysis, and assess the generalizability of the findings. The following were typically lacking: specifics about the nature of the intervention, sample size, details on how key measures were calculated, adjustment for inflation and whether there was discounting before aggregating monies from different calendar years. Only three studies provided substantial detail: namely, Lanoie and Tavenas (1996), Loisel *et al.* (2002), and DeRango *et al.* (2003), although even these lacked some information that would have been useful to the reader.

Summary and conclusions

Our two main findings from a review of the OHS intervention literature are that few workplace-based intervention studies undertake economic analyses, and the intervention studies that do undertake economic analyses present a mixed bag of methodological approaches and quality.

We have attempted to summarize and illustrate the key methodological shortcomings in order to provide insights and prescriptions for future applications in this field. Some of the issues may arise because of limited expertise in economic evaluation methodologies, others may be associated with a low priority being given to economic analysis by evaluators, and yet others relate to practical limitations of the workplace context that can prove to be a challenging hurdle. Although we have provided some preliminary recommendations, other chapters in this text explore these issues in greater detail, and present a fuller set of recommendations on how to advance the application of economic methods in the OHS field.

Chapter 4

Lessons from health technology assessment

Anthony J. Culyer and Mark Sculpher

Introduction

Economic evaluation is widely used to assist decision making in health care. The forms most commonly met are cost-effectiveness analysis (CEA) and cost–utility analysis (CUA). These methods are well-suited to one of the objectives common to many health care systems in developed countries, which is to maximize health subject to a budget constraint. One of the reasons why many societies do not rely completely on private markets for health care and health insurance is that markets are imperfect and do not always generate efficient outcomes. Another reason is that societies may have strong views on distribution of health and health care, issues that are not easily addressed through private markets alone.

The more common market imperfections in health care include the presence of professional and industrial monopolies, asymmetries of information between providers and consumers, imperfect agency relationships between health professionals and patients (and third party payers and health professionals), supplier-induced demand, externalities, incomplete markets for health care and health insurance, adverse selection, moral hazard, and the fact that individuals with limited ability to pay often have the greatest need for care (for a more complete review of the implications of these factors, see Culyer 1991). While the markets for many goods and services are characterized by the presence of some of these features, few are so thoroughly imbued with all of them. The workplace health and safety field has many of these same characteristics as health care (see the discussion in Chapter 2 for details) and, in addition, is markedly affected by the ways in which the labour market operates, which is beset by further market failures.

In light of the weaknesses of much of the economic evaluation work that has been conducted to date in workplace health and safety (see Chapter 3 for details), there is good reason to consider the lessons that can be learned from health technology assessment, where methodologies and the use of economic evaluation in policy decision making are much more advanced. Hence, in this chapter we draw on the experiences in health technology assessment to inform the use of economic evaluation in occupational health and safety (OHS), and touch on some of the problems that arise in connection with the application of these methods in health and safety interventions, especially those that differentiate their application in this field from applications in health care. We also provide a checklist to help researchers to design better studies, and to help researchers and research consumers alike to assess the quality of studies better than has usually been the case. Finally, we discuss the arguments for developing a reference case.

Economic evaluation in the policy context
Policy context in health care

As has just been noted, economic evaluation has been used widely in the health care sector as a key element in funding and formulary decisions, clinical guideline development, and other health policy planning. However, establishing the cost-effectiveness (or its absence) of various interventions in the health care setting is a costly undertaking and in general is prohibitively expensive for individual hospitals, small health regions, or even provinces like some found in Canada. For this reason, high-level arms-length bodies have emerged such as the National Institute for Health and Clinical Excellence (NICE) in England and Wales, the Pharmaceutical Benefits Advisory Committee in Australia and the Common Drug Review process in Canada, which provide evidence on the economic merits of health technologies and are intended to inform national decision making. These organizations review existing evidence related to the costs and consequences of health care interventions, and employ standard evaluation techniques in order to make recommendations to regulators, drug plans, health regions or governments (regional and national). Likewise, in a workplace health and safety context, there may be interventions of relevance to many industries, firms, and workers, but it will often be too costly for individual firms to evaluate them and the benefits of doing so will flow well beyond the confines of any individual organization. This suggests that health and safety evaluation studies have some of the characteristics of a public benefit and that those which are undertaken will often be of use to a number of organizations, particularly if such studies were to present results in a way that facilitated both a comparison with other evaluations and an assessment of generalizability of the results.

A dual purpose in the evaluation of workplace interventions

In health care, economic analyses typically take a single perspective (such as that of the payer or health care system as a whole), whereas in other contexts there is value in studies considering costs and consequences from a range of different perspectives such as those of employers, workers, workers' families, injured workers' care-givers, insurers, and public authorities. This is likely to be the case in evaluating workplace interventions.

Considering multiple perspectives highlights two possible information roles for economic evaluation. First, it serves to identify those interventions that are worth undertaking from whichever perspective is selected. This purpose is, therefore, that of helping decision makers to form a view as to whether, on balance, an intervention ought to be adopted. Secondly, evaluations can help to identify the reasons why some apparently worthwhile interventions are not adopted by highlighting the way in which the gains and losses from implementation are distributed across different groups. For example, a workplace intervention whose benefits accrue mainly to workers, but whose costs fall mainly upon employers is less likely to be implemented, even if overall benefits exceed overall costs, than one in which the benefits and costs are both realized entirely by employers. Not all evaluations of interventions will meet the criteria of a full-scale social welfare maximization exercise, since the informational requirements of such an analysis are substantial. However, they can still provide information to workers and employers that can be used in the bargaining process, thereby reducing asymmetries of information, and they can increase the information available to higher-level decision makers seeking to form an overall judgment of the worth of interventions of various kinds.

We shall assume that both information roles are equally important. The first helps to establish the social worth of interventions (and their appropriate scale), and the second helps to identify the steps that might need to be taken in order to ensure implementation, whether voluntarily or through regulation or subsidy. In addition, the second role can help identify specific distributional matters that ought to form part of the assessment of social worth seen through the lens of equity or social justice.

The methods of economic evaluation

The National Institute for Health and Clinical Excellence (NICE) in the UK, more than any other health care agency, has made the use of economic evaluation a key decision tool for public policy regarding the introduction and manner of use of health care technologies. Given the parallels between the challenges faced in the health care sector and those in OHS, there is clearly value in examining the ways in which agencies such as NICE have employed standardized economic evaluation techniques to inform the resource planning process across diverse groups (patients, care providers, insurers). We draw on their experience in the rest of this chapter.

Different types of analysis

There are broadly four kinds of economic evaluation, each of which can be found in the literature of health economics: cost–benefit analysis (CBA, sometimes called benefit–cost analysis), cost–effectiveness analysis (CEA, sometimes called cost-efficiency analysis), cost–utility analysis (CUA), and cost-minimization analysis (CMA). In addition, cost–consequence analysis (CCA) compares disaggregated costs and consequences of options without attempting to add or combine them in any way, leaving these tasks to the decision maker (see Box 4.1 for summary descriptions and Chapter 9 for details). Although CCA has generally been thought to fall short of a full economic evaluation in health care, it is often a useful precursor to a full-fledged analysis and it is a helpful framework for dealing with multiple perspectives. For the purpose of our discussion here, it suffices to say that the primary difference between the various types of economic analyses is the metric used for the key consequences (the terms 'benefit', 'outcome', and 'effect' are also used regularly in place of 'consequence').

Box 4.1 Types of economic evaluations

Cost–benefit analysis (benefit–cost analysis): compares the costs and the money-valued benefits of various alternative courses of action.

Cost-effectiveness analysis (cost-efficiency analysis): compares the opportunity costs of various alternative courses of action in terms of a common unit of outcome. Used when benefits are difficult to value monetarily, when it is socially unacceptable to do so, and when those that are measurable are not commensurable, as when the objectives of the system are in terms of health itself.

Cost–utility analysis: a close relative of cost-effectiveness analysis (and sometimes referred to as such), but which measures benefit in standardized units such as Quality-Adjusted Life-Years (QALYs). It takes its name from the use of utility type measures of outcome.

Cost-minimization analysis: a simplified form of cost-effectiveness analysis, in which cost is the dominant determining factor in a choice between alternatives, as the outcome or the value of the outcome is for practical purposes the same for each alternative.

Cost–consequence analysis: compares disaggregated costs and consequences of options without attempting to add or combine them in any way.

Although there are important differences between the different types of economic evaluation (see Sculpher *et al.* 2005), they have shared features. Each requires the calculation of present values of cost and benefit using a social discount rate. Each requires the systematic comparison of all the relevant effects of proposed alternative interventions with a view to determining:

1) which intervention, scale of intervention, or combination of interventions, produces the best outcome (either minimum cost or maximum difference between benefits and costs); or

2) the magnitude of the benefit that can result from interventions having similar costs.

Depending on the perspective of the analysis, costs falling on different affected parties (e.g., health system, patients) will be included. Each customarily uses sensitivity analysis for assessing the robustness of the conclusions in the face of variations in the assumptions and uncertainty in the evidence used. Other common characteristics are explicitness in the objectives, assumptions and methods, and consistency in the principles guiding the choice among alternatives.

Opportunity cost

Each type of economic evaluation relies on the concept of opportunity cost. Opportunity cost is the value of a resource in its most highly valued alternative use. In a world of perfect markets in which all goods are traded, opportunity costs are revealed by the market prices of resources, since these prices represent the lowest sum of money required to bid the resources away from their most highly valued possible alternative uses. Where the stringent conditions required for perfect markets are not met, opportunity costs and market prices can diverge, and true opportunity costs (shadow prices) may need to be imputed. The opportunity cost of a resource already owned by an organization is not usually revealed through a market price. The best alternative may be an alternative use within the organization; however, it is not revealed by competitive bidding between managers, but through planning processes, with the opportunity cost being elicited through discussion and judgment, without the cost necessarily being cast in terms of money.

One example of the importance of opportunity costs arises in health technology assessment when a budget-constrained health care system is considering funding a new technology, which will impose additional costs. To balance the budget an existing technology/programme will have to be removed. The aim of economic evaluation methods is to assess whether the benefits of the new technology outweigh the opportunity costs.

Opportunity costs should not be confused with transfer payments. When trades take place in a monetized economy, payments reflect the compensation required for resource owners to part with something of value. Transfer payments, on the other hand, are not made in exchange for resources and so do not measure the value of any such resources. They are merely a transfer of purchasing power from one individual or group to another. Box 4.2 identifies alternative concepts of costs and prices. Chapter 10 elaborates on these constructs. In general, opportunity cost cannot be defined independently of the decision-making context, since it involves identifying the expected consequences of alternative courses of action, and so cannot simply be read off conventional financial accounts.

Box 4.2 Alternative concepts of costs and prices

Opportunity cost: the value of a resource in its most highly valued alternative use.

Market price: the price of a resource in the market. This price may reflect the marginal value of resources embodied in the good or service if the market operates well.

Shadow price: the price a consumer is willing to pay for one more unit of a good or service. This is a reflection of the opportunity cost, but may differ from the market price if there are constraints in price and/or restrictions in supply. It is the equilibrium price in a perfect market.

Transfer payment: a transfer of purchasing power from one individual or group to another that is not a compensation for parting with the ownership of something (like a consumable item or labour). Usually made for the purpose of social equity or, as is the case with subsidies, to provide incentives for people to behave in particular ways.

Analytic perspective

'Analytic perspective' refers to the nature of the analyst's role and task in the context of an economic evaluation. One common perspective is often termed the 'social decision-making perspective'. Under the social decision-making perspective, the analyst addresses questions of concern to, and the values of, the decision maker or the organization in which s/he operates. In one form of this, the analyst plays the role of consultant, having the social decision maker as client. In another, the organization has its objectives and constraints explicitly defined, for example, by a higher policymaking body, and these can guide the analyst. Another analytic perspective is termed the societal perspective.

This usually entails the analyst defining a more or less broad concept of social welfare and making explicit the social value judgments involved in so doing. With this approach there is the risk that the analyst adopts criteria that are seen as irrelevant by real world decision makers. Other perspectives are more specific, for example, those of the owners of businesses, or (not the same thing) the managers of businesses, or unionized workers, or all workers, or workers' families, or third party payers (such as workers' compensation boards). The things that count as benefits and costs, and that get caught up in externalities, can vary significantly depending on which viewpoint is adopted. A major guiding principle of all economic evaluations is consequently that the analytic perspective must be stated explicitly so that readers can assess for themselves the consequences by way of inclusion or exclusion of the various possible effects for the decisions informed by the analysis.

Value judgments

All forms of economic evaluation require value judgments. The choice of perspective itself commits the analyst to particular value judgments. In addition, the analyst needs to make other critical choices, all of which involve value judgments, some of which may be more specific and precise than the ones directly or indirectly implied by the values embodied in the chosen perspective. For example, a perspective emphasizing health may specifically entail selecting the QALY as an outcome; a perspective emphasizing social cost may specifically select costs falling on the public sector; and a general requirement for equity may need specific decisions relating to the weighting of consequences based on whether a dollar is gained/lost by stockholders or workers. A decision to treat monetary consequences with equal weight regardless of who is experiencing the loss or gain is not a means of escaping the value issue. On the contrary, it is to make a very specific value judgment, which is that it is appropriate to value each dollar of consequence equally.

Evaluation of interventions: the health technology assessment experience

In the health care field the word 'technology' is used quite broadly to refer to 'a means of accomplishing something.' It includes the use of health care technologies such as scanners, prescription drugs, bed rest, and watchful waiting. Although less frequently encountered there, it applies also to the evaluation of technologies of governance and managerial arrangement. Counterparts in OHS might be the use of machine guards or ergonomically designed workstations and the use of OHS management systems.

Health technology assessment (HTA) has had an increasingly prominent position in health care policy internationally. Although much HTA research has been funded and published since the late 1960s, it was not until the mid-1990s that it gained a formal foothold in policymaking. In the last decade, many health care systems in developed countries have decided to inform decisions about the adoption of new health interventions by use of economic evaluation of the clinical and epidemiological evidence. While these requirements have been applied principally to pharmaceuticals, the range of technologies requiring such evidence before adoption has tended to be broadened over time (for example, public health interventions were added to NICE's range of responsibilities in 2005). A formal requirement for economic analysis to support reimbursement or coverage began in the public systems of Ontario, Canada (Ministry of Health 1994) and Australia (Commonwealth Department of Health, Housing and Community Services 1992), but have since spread widely (Hjelmgren *et al.* 2001). Australia, Belgium, Canada, England and Wales, Israel and Scotland have all published guidelines for economic evaluations as inputs into decisions about coverage and reimbursement (Tarn and Smith 2005).

The methodology of economic evaluation has developed rapidly over the last 40 years. The research methods used for health care system decision making today are much more sophisticated than those employed in the past. Early economic evaluations commonly assumed (often only implicitly) that the objective of health care was to maximize gross domestic product. This may be illustrated by an analysis of the economic consequences of preventing the birth of babies with Down's syndrome through screening (Hagard and Carter 1976). In this study, the benefits of screening were seen in terms of avoiding the costs of caring for and educating a child with Down's syndrome, implicitly assuming that there was no intrinsic or even human capital benefit to a life (Culyer 1987). As noted in Chapter 2, the naïve human capital approach to valuing the benefits of health care fails to recognize that individuals value health for reasons other than the productive potential it generates and they value lives for reasons other than the gross domestic product each life may manufacture (net, of course, of human maintenance costs) (Mishan 1971; Blades *et al.* 1987).

For much of the subsequent period it became increasingly clear that there were serious tensions between the principles of standard welfare economics (essentially the societal perspective described above), and a more flexible and decision-oriented perspective on evaluative research towards which many health economists were leaning. Although standard welfare economics gives clear guidance on what is meant by efficiency, how costs and benefits should be measured, what perspective should be taken, and whether the adoption of a new health technology improves social welfare, it has strong normative underpinnings which require leaps of faith to accept (Sculpher *et al.* 2005).

Essentially, welfare economics has a number of significant and controversial implications for evaluation in health care. The first is that heath care programmes should be evaluated in the same way as other programmes. The concern here is that standard welfare economics relies on a particular construct of efficiency known as a 'potential Pareto improvement' measured by a compensation test like 'can the gainers compensate the losers—either in theory or practice—and still retain a net gain?' The criteria are meant to ensure that there are no utility losses after suitable compensation, only utility gains, since the principles of welfare economics do not allow one to make a direct comparison of the value of utility losses to one individual with the value of gains to another (see Box 4.3 for more detailed definitions). An outcome where there are some utility gainers and no net utility losers is considered to mark an unambiguous gain in social welfare.

The standard welfare economics approach is not well-suited to addressing matters, such as whether an intervention improves life expectancy or health, which is the standard clinician's or health policy decision maker's question. It focuses on the much more obscure matter (from clinician's or policymaker's viewpoint) of whether the intervention improves utility. The clinician's or health policy decision maker's approach is, however, the basis of outcome metrics known as health-related quality of life (HRQL) measures and many

Box 4.3 Pareto constructs

Pareto criterion of efficiency: An allocation is considered efficient if there is no way to reallocate resources (with compensation to losers) such that one or more individuals is made better off without making someone else worse off in terms of their net utility. This is a very restrictive concept of efficiency, since it limits the types of reallocation that can be made.

Potential Pareto improvement: This is measured by a compensation test like 'could the gainers in principle compensate the losers and still retain a net gain?' It is a less stringent criterion than the Pareto criterion of efficiency, since it allows net utility losses and gains.

health economists essentially adopt an approach that is based on the idea that health services exist primarily to create health rather than utility.

A second controversial aspect of welfare economics is an implicit view that the current distribution of income is, if not optimal, then at least acceptable (Pauly 1995) and that the distributive impact of a decision based on economic evaluation is or ought to be negligible. Other controversies include the conditions of rationality and consistency that are required for individuals to maximize their utility, which have been shown to be violated in most choice situations (Machina 1987), and the problem of second best (e.g., Ng 1983), whereby first best solutions in a second best world (i.e., a situation where only some of the conditions of the ideal solution are met) may actually represent a reduction in social welfare as defined by the potential Pareto criterion.

There is an alternative to the standard welfare economics approach to economic evaluation in health care. In the United Kingdom and elsewhere, an approach described as 'extra welfarist' (Culyer 1991) has provided the methodological foundations of economic evaluation in health care (see Box 4.4 for details). It is a version of the social decision-making perspective and uses CUA, rather than CBA. It is based on an exogenously defined objective (such as population health maximization) and an exogenously determined budget constraint for health care. The efficiency problem is thereby transformed into another constrained maximization problem (i.e., how to maximize the amount of incremental health produced by a given budget). This pragmatic approach is well-suited to partial analyses that assume that there are few significant repercussions of health care decisions beyond the health sector itself. Correspondingly, it is not well-suited to the analysis of intersectoral choices, where the outcome measures will typically be different and pose major issues of relative valuation, and where opportunity costs may become difficult to identify.

Box 4.4 Welfarism and extra-welfarism

Welfarism in economics: the welfare economics approach is based on individual utilities and preferences, expressed through market or shadow prices, as the basis for the evaluation of efficiency.

Extra-welfarism: the extra-welfarist approach in health care views health as the maximand, rather than utility or social welfare. The concept of 'health' may or may not be based on the preferences of the target population.

One of the implications of using the extra-welfarist approach in health care is that it facilitates a multi-disciplinary outlook to the research, requiring the identification and synthesizing of relevant clinical and other evidence, mathematical models to characterize the natural history of a given disease and the effects of interventions, the definition of measurement and valuation of health gain, and quantification and valuation of the resource implications.

Hence, major contributions to this research are made by various disciplines including clinical science, cognitive psychology, decision science, epidemiology, medical statistics, and operations research, in addition to economics.

Differences in the sources and treatment of bias

A major difference between the information available for an economic appraisal in health care compared to that available for workplace intervention evaluation is the character and treatment of bias. In evaluating the effectiveness of medical technologies (in particular drugs), randomization is often used in clinical trials to control for potential confounding factors, whereas this is rarely possible in workplace intervention evaluation. Both the location and the size of workplace evaluations rarely permit randomization. Thus, it becomes necessary to anticipate confounders as best as may be possible—for example by measuring them explicitly in observational studies for subsequent multivariate analysis or, minimally, by exercising well-informed judgment. The careful use of sensitivity analysis often enables the identification of omitted variables or poorly measured ones, as well as giving an indication of the extent to which the changes in outcome attributed to the intervention are robust.

A second source of bias relates to the decisions made by the analyst about the costs and consequences that are to be measured, how one is traded off against another, and how to add them up across different individuals (see Chapter 2 for a more detailed discussion of these issues). These matters may be of less concern in health care because costs and consequences are less often distributed across such varied categories of stakeholders. In general, there is no right answer to these questions. The answers are likely to be controversial and raise major questions of policy, politics, ethics, and public acceptability. This is not an argument for helplessness, for the identification of such issues is an important part of the decision-making process and any measurement of relevant dimensions will usually be helpful. The conclusion, therefore, is that analysts ought to be open and explicit about the value content of their analyses, to face up directly to the challenges that rival values might pose and, whenever useful, to subject value judgments to the same kind of sensitivity analysis that is recommended for design attributes. The merit of this approach is in identifying value judgments that do or do not, as the case may be, affect the major results of the analysis, and providing decision makers with such evidence about values that may have a bearing on their decisions.

A brief description of current key methodological guidance

As economic evaluation has become more widely undertaken and formally used in health care decision making, much energy has gone into developing methodological guidelines for researchers. In general, these can be divided into two categories: guidelines developed as a scientific statement of good practice in the field, and guidelines issued by particular decision-making agencies to define the approach to economic evaluation deemed to be appropriate in their jurisdiction.

With regard to scientific statements of good practice, two particularly authoritative documents are worth noting. The first is a widely known text-book, *Methods for the Economic Evaluation of Health Care Programmes*, now in its third edition (Drummond *et al.* 2005). A consistently important element of this book since its first edition has been the inclusion of a methods checklist for critiquing economic evaluation studies. An adaptation of this is reproduced in Table 4.1. Essentially, the checklist focuses on the need for clear description of a study and the use of those methods that are considered to be good practice in economic evaluation. The list emphasizes key aspects of a sound evaluation such as explicitly stating the perspective used in the analysis, using incremental analysis, discounting future costs and consequences, and giving adequate attention to uncertainty in the estimates and to the implications of omitted relevant variables. The need for such a list became clear from reviews of earlier evaluations, most of which were deficient in many more than just one or two respects.

The second document was developed by a multi-disciplinary panel convened by the US Public Health Service and published in 1996 (Gold *et al.* 1996). It also provides a description of methods issues and recommendations for good practice. This text is more prescriptive in its recommendations than Drummond *et al.* (2005). It also introduced the idea of a reference case, a concept to which we return later. Key aspects of the US Panel's recommendations were:

◆ *A societal perspective should be taken*. In part, this relates to resource costs, and requires that costs falling both on a health care budget and outside it should be included in analyses. Importantly, it requires inclusion of costs such as travel, which are borne by patients and time costs borne by relatives caring for patients. The US Panel took an innovative view on the treatment of the productivity effects of health care interventions. They concluded that,

Table 4.1 A checklist for assessing economic evaluations based on Drummond *et al.* (2005).

---

1. Was a well-defined question posed in answerable form?

    1.1 Did the study examine both costs and effects of the intervention?

    1.2 Did the study involve a comparison of alternatives?

    1.3 Was a perspective for the analysis stated and was the study placed in any particular decision-making context?

2. Was an adequately comprehensive description of the competing alternatives given? (i.e., can you tell who did what to whom, where, and how often for each option?)

    2.1 Were all relevant alternatives included?

    2.2 Was a *do-nothing* alternative considered? If not, were there good reasons why it was inappropriate?

3. Was the effectiveness or ineffectiveness of the intervention established?

    3.1 Was this done through a randomized controlled trial? If so, did the trial protocol reflect what would happen in regular practice? If not, how were confounding factors controlled?

    3.2 Were effectiveness data collected and summarized through a systematic review of studies? If so, were the search strategy and rules for inclusion or exclusion outlined?

    3.3 Were observational data or assumptions used to establish effectiveness? If so, what were the potential biases in the results?

    3.4 If the study was an efficacy study, was any attempt made to assess its generalizability?

4. Were all the important and relevant costs and consequences for each alternative identified?

    4.1 Was the range wide enough for the research question at hand?

    4.2 Did the range include material useful to all relevant perspectives?

    4.3 Were all relevant costs (labour, capital, as well as operating costs) included?

    4.4 Were all relevant consequences (for all parties potentially affected, whether or not engaged in the workplace) included?

5. Were costs and consequences measured accurately in appropriate physical units (e.g., hours of nursing time, number of physician visits, work days gained or lost, life-years gained or lost, effects on workers' families)?

    5.1 Were the sources of resource utilization described and justified?

    5.2 Were any possibly significant costs or consequences omitted from consideration or, if identified, not measured well? What weight did they carry in the subsequent analysis?

    5.3 Were there any special circumstances (e.g., joint use of resources) that made measurement difficult? Were these issues handled appropriately rather than being simply ignored?

Continued

Table 4.1 (continued) A checklist for assessing economic evaluations based on Drummond *et al.* (2005).

6. Were costs and consequences valued credibly?

    6.1 Were the sources of all values clearly identified? (Possible sources include market values, worker or employer preferences and views through surveys, policymakers' views and health professionals' judgments.)

    6.2 Where market values were absent (e.g., value of family care-givers' time) or did not reflect actual values (such as clinic space donated at a reduced rate), were adjustments made to approximate market values?

    6.3 Was the valuation of consequences appropriate for the question posed (i.e., was the appropriate type of analysis (CEA, CUA, CBA) selected)?

7. Were costs and consequences adjusted for differential timing?

    7.1 Were costs and consequences occurring in the future discounted to their present values?

    7.2 Was any justification given for the discount rate(s) used?

8. Was an incremental analysis of costs and consequences of alternatives performed?

    8.1 Were the additional (incremental) costs generated by one alternative over another compared with the additional effects, benefits, or utilities generated?

9. Was allowance made for uncertainty in the estimation of costs and consequences?

    9.1 If workplace level data on costs or consequences were available, were appropriate statistical analyses performed?

    9.2 If a sensitivity analysis was employed, was justification provided for the ranges or distributions of values (for key study parameters), and the form of sensitivity analysis used?

    9.3 Were the authors' conclusions sensitive to the uncertainty in the results, as quantified by the statistical and/or sensitivity analysis?

10. Did the presentation and discussion of study results include all issues of concern to users?

    10.1 Were the conclusions of the analysis based on some overall index or ratio of costs to consequences (e.g., cost-effectiveness ratio)? If so, was the index interpreted intelligently or in a mechanistic fashion? If not, was any guidance offered as to how decision makers might seek to make an overall judgment of effectiveness or cost-effectiveness?

    10.2 Were the results compared with those of others who have investigated the same or similar question? If so, were allowances made for potential differences in study methodology?

    10.3 Did the study discuss the generalizability of the results to other settings, workplaces, or industrial sectors?

    10.4 Did the study allude to, or take account of, other important factors in the choice or decision under consideration (e.g., distribution of costs and consequences, political constraints, or relevant ethical issues)?

Table 4.1 (continued) A checklist for assessing economic evaluations based on Drummond *et al.* (2005)

10.5 Did the study discuss issues of implementation, such as the feasibility of adopting the preferred programme given existing financial or other constraints, and whether any freed resources could be redeployed to other worthwhile programmes?
10.6 Did the study involve key stakeholders at relevant phases, such as the choice of intervention and comparators, selection of research question, selection of workplaces, choice of value judgments (such as the weights to be attached to dissimilar consequences), the concept of equity to be used, and the ease of implementation in the short, medium and long term?

in part, these would already be captured by the valuation of health (they recommended use of the QALY as the outcome measure), while residual productivity effects (such as those falling on the wider community through, for example, reduced taxation) ought to be explicitly included. The choice of a societal perspective also implies the inclusion of all health and non-health effects (both positive and negative) to intended recipients and others. Evaluative studies of workplace interventions have typically left the issue of perspective implicit. Some appear largely to view evaluation through a worker's lens and other through an employer's lens. Virtually none has systematically taken a more comprehensive view.

♦ *Health effects should be expressed in terms of QALYs.* This is a measure of health that incorporates the effects of interventions on both mortality (through changes in survival duration) and morbidity (through effects on health-related quality of life). The US Panel thus embraced CUA/CEA as the appropriate analytic paradigm. In the workplace intervention evaluation literature there is no convention regarding the measurement (or even the relevance) of health effects, other than through its impact on productivity.

♦ *Effectiveness estimates from best-designed and least-biased sources should be used.* Reflecting the typical limitations and heterogeneity of the clinical evidence base available for economic evaluation, this recommendation leans towards using best available evidence. The point can also apply to sources of non-clinical evidence such as resource costs. Other guidelines have emphasized the importance of incorporating all evidence given the hazards of selecting best evidence (National Institute for Clinical Excellence 2004). As noted earlier, effectiveness evidence is more likely to be biased in various ways when based on data observed in workplaces. Assessment of bias or the quality and generalizability of evidence is rarely addressed in any systematic way in workplace intervention evaluations.

- *Comparison should be made with existing practice and (if necessary) viable low-cost alternatives.* Comparator technologies (minimally the status quo) are always necessary. However, decisions about the range of options to compare within an economic evaluation are central to the appropriate specification of an economic evaluation to guide decision making. Leaving out a relevant option can result in highly misleading results. Comparators are rarely used in workplace evaluations and, where they are, they are rarely described explicitly.

- *One-way and multi-way sensitivity analysis (for important parameters) should be undertaken.* It is recognized that all analyses will be characterized by uncertainty about key elements of evidence. Sensitivity analysis is, as has been seen, a means of exploring the extent to which the conclusions of a study are robust to the changes in the value of key inputs. In analyzing workplace interventions, problems of incompatible values and political differences are likely to loom more prominently than in the case of the clinical literature, so sensitivity analysis ought also to be used to test the dependence of the conclusions on controversial value judgments. Sensitivity analysis is virtually unknown in the evaluative literature of workplace interventions.

There are now many methods guidelines issued by decision-making agencies. These have recently been surveyed by the International Society for Pharmacoeconomics and Outcomes Research (Tarn and Smith 2005). They display considerable variation, both in terms of how prescriptive they are and in their specific recommendations. Table 4.2 illustrates the variation using the example of recommendations for the selection of options for comparison.

The National Institute for Health and Clinical Excellence (NICE) in the UK issued methods guidelines for analyses being undertaken as inputs to its Technology Appraisal Programme (National Institute for Clinical Excellence 2004). The guidelines set out the requirements for economic evaluation based on the characteristics of the decisions that the organization is charged to make and the specific constraints under which it operates. NICE's recommendations are prescriptive and go beyond those of the US Panel in a number of respects. Notable recommendations are:

- The use of systematic reviews to identify all appropriate evidence on effectiveness for economic evaluation.

- The use of a validated generic measure of health-related quality of life as a basis for formulating the morbidity component of QALYs.

- Restrictions on the types of costs and consequences to a set deemed relevant by policymakers in the Department of Health (the perspective taken is essentially that of public sector managers).

Table 4.2 Variation in recommendations for comparator technologies. Reproduced from Sculpher and Drummond (2006), based on data from Tarn and Smith (2005).

Recommended comparator technology	No. of guidelines
Most commonly used alternative	8
Existing technology, most effective or minimum practice	2
Existing or most effective technology	1
A justified alternative technology	1
Both existing technology and no treatment	2
Most common technology, least costly, no treatment	1
Most common technology, most effective, least costly, and no treatment	2
Most common technology, least costly, and most effective	1
Most likely technology to be displaced	1
Most efficient technology, most effective, and do nothing	2
All relevant comparators	2
Most effective technology and no treatment	1
Not clear or unspecific	3

- ◆ The use of probabilistic sensitivity analysis which simultaneously assesses the implications of uncertainty in all parameters within an evaluation and allows this to be presented in terms of the probability that a particular option is the most cost-effective, conditional on how much the health care system is willing to pay for a QALY (Claxton *et al.* 2005).

Case for a reference case

A key feature of both the US Panel's statement of good practice in economic evaluation and NICE's 2004 methodological guidance is the definition of a reference case. The purpose of a reference case is to provide consistency in methods used in all evaluations regardless of the disease areas or technologies being evaluated.

The need for consistency is a response to two important features of economic evaluation in health care. The first is the lack of consensus about some areas of methodology. These include the choice of study type (e.g., CUA vs. CBA), the source of preference and value data (e.g., patients versus the general public), the approach to describing health states for valuation, and the inclusion of future costs that appear to be unrelated to the intervention of interest, but are incurred because life expectancy is extended by the intervention. By taking a position on each of these, a reference case can be seen as either defining an authoritative view about the most appropriate method, or as simply selecting one approach in order to avoid unhelpful variability between analyses. The second feature of consistency between studies relates to pragmatic uncertainty. This relates to the need for decision makers to specify their preferred methods, in particular as they embody political or value content in the policy context in which the analysis is to be used. For example, they may wish to be explicit about what they consider to be the appropriate cost perspective and the types of equity issues to be considered.

Stipulating a reference case does not preclude analysts undertaking other types of analysis (e.g., different approaches to health valuation). However, such alternative approaches would need to be undertaken in addition to the reference case and should be justified on the basis of potential shortcomings of the reference case in a specific context.

Would a reference case be helpful to guide researchers undertaking economic evaluations in the context of OHS interventions? It is clear that there is even greater lack of consensus about appropriate evaluation methods for workplace interventions than in health care (see Chapter 3). As a result, the vast majority of studies do not meet the minimal quality requirements in the checklist and it is virtually impossible to make comparisons between the effectiveness, let alone the cost-effectiveness, of alternative interventions reported in different studies. There is, however, an important difference between work-related interventions and health care: there is no single decision maker (such as a reimbursement agency in health care) for whom the analysis is undertaken, and who might be perceived as having an authoritative set of objectives and constraints that ought to be reflected in the methods chosen for the economic analysis. Rather, policy changes relating to workplace health and safety are more likely to be based on interactions between key stakeholders. These include employers (who are likely to incur much of the cost of interventions and only a portion of benefit in terms of productivity changes), as well as labour representatives, workers' compensation and insurance boards, government and regulators. Therefore, any reference case in this area would need to reflect the multiple perspectives that may be had in any particular decision context. It would be appropriate for the reference case to stipulate a societal perspective on costs, health effects and other effects that would indicate what should be done considering the net cost and effects on everyone. However, it would also be necessary for the reference case to require that analyses include estimates of the distribution of costs and effects between stakeholders, which would provide both the various parties affected with a basis for policy negotiations and political decision makers with a basis for making an overall assessment.

Conclusions

The way in which the labour market determines decisions about health and safety is fraught with imperfections. This suggests that a reliance on market mechanisms alone is unlikely to deliver the optimal degree of prevention, protection, or compensation. The labour market is also the classic setting for political conflict between labour and employers. It can generate profound inequalities in society, which many may regard as inherently and deeply unjust. For such reasons, if economic analysis is to be used to replace or substitute for the market mechanism it needs to offer a methodology that does not replicate these imperfections, and not one that introduces new and no less unsatisfactory biases. One way may be to simulate the operation of a perfect market (this is, in essence, the objective of economic evaluations done according to the customary rules of neoclassical welfare economics), and the other is to postulate specific objectives and constraints that are appropriate to the sector and problem at hand (this is, in essence, one manifestation of the social decision-making perspective).

We do not advocate either in preference to the other here. However, what we do suggest is that analysts ought to be as explicit as possible about the key structural elements of their analyses, their sources of evidence and the values embodied in their interpretations of findings. We have provided a checklist based upon one commonly used in health technology assessment. It serves to assist those wishing to undertake well-designed workplace intervention studies with economic components, and those wishing to compare or evaluate existing studies.

Chapter 5

Lessons from the literature on valuing reductions in physical risk

Richard Cookson and Peter Dorman

Introduction

The economic literature on valuing reductions in physical risk (or 'valuing safety', for short) concerns attempts to value the prevention of injury and disease in economic evaluations. There are several general literature reviews (Viscusi 1993; Beattie *et al.* 1998a) and textbooks (Jones-Lee 1989; Viscusi 1992; Dorman 1996) on the topic. A more comprehensive review from which this chapter was developed is also available as a working paper (Cookson and Dorman 2008).

Economic evaluations of occupational health and safety (OHS) interventions typically focus on the cost savings associated with preventing occupational injury and disease from an employer's perspective, for example, via increased worker productivity, lower health care costs, and lower workers' compensation payments (Niven 2002). The valuing safety literature takes a different approach. It focuses on the human costs of injury and disease in terms of harm to individual well-being and examines how individuals value reductions in physical risk for themselves. It aims to quantify the value of intangible human outcomes, such as pain and suffering, as well as tangible financial outcomes such as loss of livelihood. It aims to value all such outcomes in monetary terms so that they can be compared with the costs and consequences of other policy interventions under consideration. It is not concerned with estimating the effectiveness of OHS interventions in terms of lives saved, or injuries prevented, or days of pain, grief and suffering avoided. Thus, it falls under the category of cost–benefit analysis (CBA), rather than cost-effectiveness analysis (CEA) or cost–utility analysis (CUA).

The standard approach focuses on small changes in physical risks. The economist analyzes the trade-offs that individuals are willing to make (or are imputed to make) between physical risk and wealth or other non-health benefits (e.g., time, convenience, consumption of goods and services, working conditions). Empirical estimates of such trade-offs use either revealed preference data from real market transactions (in particular, imputed wage-risk trade-offs) or expressed preference data from questionnaires that ask people to make hypothetical trade-offs. The resulting monetary valuations can be thought of as values of a statistical life (VSL). They do not reflect the value of saving an identified person from imminent death but the value of a small reduction in the probability of a single fatality amongst a large number of individuals, which more closely reflects the reality of most OHS interventions (see Box 5.1 for a stylized example).

Estimates of the VSL started appearing in the 1970s, with most of the work originating from labour economics and transport economics. It is perhaps ironic that economic evaluations of OHS interventions have tended to ignore this literature, even though so much of it originated from the study of work-place risk. The empirical literature on valuing safety mushroomed in the 1990s, with a substantial increase in both the volume and breadth of empirical studies, particularly those using the theory of expressed preferences (discussed later in this chapter), including studies in other sub-disciplines of economics (e.g., environmental economics and health economics). The literature on expressed preferences has borrowed ideas and techniques from psychology and sociology, and has increasingly become a multi-disciplinary enterprise.

Why value human outcomes?

An answer to the practical question of whether to focus on financial or human outcomes is likely to depend primarily on the perspective of the evaluation, i.e., which individuals and/or organizations are to be the main users of the

Box 5.1 An example of calculating the value of statistical life

Consider the following simplified scenario: 100,000 workers benefit from an OHS intervention that reduces the probability of any worker dying in the next year by two in 100,000. Each worker is willing to pay a maximum of $50 for this improvement, directly out of pocket or through lower wages. Thus, the group's total maximum willingness to pay is $50 × 100,000 = $5,000,000. Dividing the total maximum willingness to pay by the expected number of deaths prevented (i.e., two) yields a value of statistical life in this setting of $2,500,000. If the total cost of the intervention was $4,000,000 then the prevention would be considered worthwhile, and workers would be better off by $1,000,000, or $10 each.

results of the evaluation? To caricature somewhat, financial outcomes may be of primary interest to a firm. This is not to deny that firms may be interested in measuring human outcomes (as well as in valuing them), especially insofar as these have important secondary effects on financial outcomes, including long-term financial outcomes of intangible assets such as reputation and trust among employees and consumers.

From the perspective of the individuals directly affected by OHS interventions, human outcomes are likely to be of primary interest, in addition to loss of future earnings and consumption. From a public sector perspective (e.g., a health and safety regulator, or the government as a whole) human outcomes may also be of considerable interest in their own right because saving lives and improving health and well-being are themselves specific public policy goals. To give somewhat stark examples, an exclusive focus on financial outcomes would imply that it is not worth saving the lives of retired or long-term unemployed individuals who are not economically productive, and that saving the lives of high-wage workers is more beneficial than saving the lives of low-wage workers, since the latter make a lower contribution to economic output at market prices. Faced with a series of somewhat unpalatable ethical implications of this kind, which violate both the assumptions of standard welfare economics and the principles of distributive justice, the human capital approach has fallen from favour among professional economists and long ago ceased to be recommended as best practice within the discipline (see Chapter 2 for a detailed discussion of concerns related to the human capital approach). Box 5.2 provides a description of the three main approaches to valuing safety in monetary terms.

The human outcomes approach, based on the value of life to the individual rather than the value of the individual's livelihood to the wider economy, has generally led to higher estimates of the monetary value of a life, especially since an allowance for lost output to the economy is often added to the human outcome values.

Welfare economics and human outcomes

Welfare economics is the starting point for economic analysis. It proposes that: 1) individuals possess preferences that can be described mathematically by utility functions conforming to certain logical rules; 2) these functions are complete over all potential outcomes; 3) these functions uniquely determine individual behaviour and are derivable from observations of behaviour; and 4) these functions constitute the only acceptable basis for ascribing value to actions or outcomes.

Box 5.2 Three approaches to valuing safety in monetary terms

There are three methods for valuing safety in monetary terms:

1) the human capital approach;
2) the revealed preference approach;
3) the expressed preference approach (contingent valuation and relative valuation).

The latter two are both willingness to pay methods.

Human capital approach views increases in human capital (a stock of productive skills determined by ability, educational attainment, and health) or prevention of reductions in it as the principal outcome of OHS interventions. Essentially, health is valued only because it allows individuals to be productive. The approach neglects any benefits that are not work-related, such as the intrinsic value of improved health or freedom from pain, and the associated enjoyment of leisure time. The human capital approach values only financial outcomes.

Revealed preference approach involves inferring the value of safety from individuals' actual choices in the marketplace, primarily from the premium workers require in compensation for higher risks. The revealed preference approach values human outcomes.

Expressed or *stated preference approach* involves directly asking individuals about their trade-offs between income and safety, or between different types of health risks. The traditional approach is to ask individuals for their maximum willingness to pay for increased safety, or the minimum monetary payment they require to forgo it. This version of the expressed preference approach is known as *contingent valuation*, since it is a method for eliciting valuations from individuals, contingent on a hypothetical market scenario. A second approach is to ask individuals for their relative valuations of one health risk against another, such as fatal versus non-fatal risk or risk from one hazard rather than another. The resulting *relative valuations* provide one or more marker monetary values to assist with deriving monetary values for other risks. The expressed preference approach also values human outcomes.

Willingness to pay and accept

In welfare economics, the choices people make are usually classified as willingness to pay (WTP) or willingness to accept (WTA). In the first case an individual wishes to acquire a benefit, and WTP is measured by the maximum amount s/he would pay for it. In the second an individual is asked to part with a benefit, and WTA is the minimum amount of compensation required if the benefit is to be relinquished voluntarily. The only difference in value between WTP and WTA would stem from the difference in initial utility, higher for WTA than WTP, all else being equal. Since utility is measured in monetary equivalents, and given the assumption of diminishing marginal utility of income for a given individual, it is expected that WTA is greater than WTP even though utility would be unchanged in either case. This is because there is higher utility associated with having the benefit initially (and being paid to give it up); hence, a given amount of utility will correspond to a larger sum of money, and vice versa. Assuming the value of the benefit is small relative to total utility, however, this difference should also be small.

These assumptions play an important role in economic theory. First, they make it possible to apply values derived in WTP contexts to WTA contexts, and vice versa. Indeed, without this it would be difficult to speak of the VSL, even for a given individual and a given risk factor. This is particularly important to bear in mind when considering labour-market studies, as we will see shortly. Secondly, these assumptions also underpin the formulation of economic efficiency as applied to the allocation of benefits such as reduced risk of injury or death. A potential Pareto improvement occurs whenever such a reduction can be achieved for a cost below the corresponding WTA/WTP measure of benefits. The idea here is that it will then hypothetically be possible for the gainers from a policy change to compensate the losers, still leaving at least one individual better off and nobody worse off. However, if WTA could diverge significantly from WTP then judgments of economic efficiency would be contingent on the initial allocation of the benefit.

Compensating wage differentials in the labour market

A particular application of utility-based risk analysis draws on data from the labour market. It is assumed that it is costly to provide safer working conditions, so that as risk increases, all else being equal, so does profit. In the labour market, workers make offers based on their utility from income and risk which have the property that, for any given worker, greater risk must be offset by a greater wage to maintain a particular level of utility. Employers make wage offers based on the expectation that any reduction in risk must be offset by a reduction in wages, if a given level of profit is to be maintained, other things being equal. Equilibrium occurs where the wage-risk trade-off is identical between workers and employers (i.e., the change in risk has exactly the same monetary value for both). Note that this logic depends on the assumption that increments of risk are increasingly disliked by workers (i.e., the marginal disutility of risk is increasing), while increments of safety are increasingly costly for employers to provide (i.e., the marginal cost of safety is increasing).

The implication of this analysis is that firms with greater difficulty in making work safer (e.g., roofing companies) would reach labour-market equilibrium at higher levels of risk. Similarly, workers with a diminished tolerance for risk would, all things being equal, reach equilibrium at lower levels of risk. Furthermore, there are efficiency gains to be had by properly matching relatively risk-tolerant workers with employers who face relatively greater costs of OHS.

The preceding model of safety determination has three significant implications. First, it yields the property that in equilibrium, all else being equal, workers in dangerous jobs are no worse off than those in safer jobs. This is because workers are fully compensated for the risk they face; they receive an increment in their wage that leaves them at the same level of utility they would otherwise be at. Second, it identifies a level of risk in the workplace that is seen as efficient in equilibrium. At this level, the marginal cost to the employer of reducing risk is exactly equal to the marginal benefit to the worker of having it reduced. Third, and for our purposes most important, it permits an estimation of the worker's implicit value of health or life. Assuming that workers are arrayed across a range of firms with different costs of safety, and assuming that they bring the same underlying utility functions to their choice of employment, the value of health impairments can be deduced from the estimated wage-risk trade-offs arrived at in the market.

This portrayal of labour markets is not broadly accepted by other disciplines, and it has attracted its share of critics among economists as well. There are several potential difficulties. First, the labour market may not equilibrate in the manner specified by the model. Excess supply is the characteristic of most labour markets that have been studied (Solow 1990), but the model under consideration reaches equilibrium where supply equals demand.

Second, in practice the most attractive employments also tend to be the best paid. Alternative employments available to a given worker do not typically provide an equivalent level of utility. Rather, workers queue for desirable jobs offering greater pay or work amenities. Those who get such jobs are better off than those who do not. If dangerous jobs are, on average, less desirable than safe ones, the market wage-risk trade-off will understate the utility trade-off. Indeed, there may even be a negative trade-off if dangerous jobs are so much worse than less dangerous jobs that they also pay lower wages.

Third, workers may not accept the working conditions as provided by the employer at the point at which an employment agreement is struck. This may be because workers expect (correctly or otherwise) that they will be able to alter these conditions, or because they believe that the law (which has rejected the assumption of risk doctrine for more than 100 years) will protect them. In any case, in the laws typically in force in industrialized countries, workers do not and cannot legally accept many of the risks they actually face at work.

Fourth, there is little direct evidence that employers perceive a wage cost associated with failure to provide safer working conditions. Textbooks used to train safety managers, for instance, go into great detail on productivity and insurance costs stemming from accidents, but they do not claim that employers will have to pay increased wage compensation for greater risk (Dorman 1996).

Fifth, the model assumes full information on both sides. In practice, the extent of risk, particularly that which is either of low probability or delayed in its effect, is not known. In addition, there is typically information asymmetry; employers know the risks better than their workers do, and have an incentive to conceal their knowledge.

Sixth, if the model is correct, there is nothing to be gained by workers demanding government regulation beyond the provision of accurate information. This can be seen by the efficiency properties of equilibrium risk; at any other level of risk the wage adjustment forced on to employers would leave workers worse off than before. Yet the history of occupational safety and health policy is one of constant agitation by workers for more assertive regulation.

Seventh, the scenario is implicitly a one-shot game played between a worker, or a set of workers, and an employer. Most economic theory prior to the 1980s was naïve game theory in this sense. During the past two decades, however, the use of game-theoretic methods has flourished in economics. It is clear that a repeated game is a better characterization of the determination of wages and risk, since employees can be regarded as recontracting over time. Whether the properties of a correctly specified repeated game would be the same as of those in a one-shot game is currently unknown, since such a model has not been analyzed.

Eighth, the model is built upon the utility propositions presented earlier, but there is empirical evidence that belies these propositions.

A final point has to do with the emphasis placed on worker choice. The model presumes that workers face a range of jobs that are approximately equal to them in utility terms. Thus, the wage increment reflects the amount workers are willing to accept (WTA) to incur added risk. To the extent that this is correct, and given the substantial differences in the literature between WTA and WTP for identical risks, researchers should be cautioned against using labour-market studies to derive values to be used in contexts in which WTP is the appropriate measure rather than WTA, such as investments in improved health care facilities (see Glossary for a more detailed discussion of WTP and WTA).

An alternative theoretical approach

The empirical literature using revealed preferences from labour-market data remains closely tied to the standard theory of welfare economics. Since the 1990s, however, the empirical literature using expressed preference data has borrowed heavily from psychology and sociology, and in so doing has at times departed somewhat from standard welfare economics and developed more sophisticated methods of measuring strength of preference. For example, focus group methods are sometimes used to help respondents arrive at more considered preferences. Some techniques include asking hypothetical questions that invite respondents to adopt the perspective of a citizen or policymaker acting on behalf of a group of people, rather than the perspective of a consumer making decisions on their own behalf. Although no definitive alternative theoretical framework has been developed to justify these departures, they may broadly be defended in terms of a 'decision-making' or 'extra-welfarist' approach to economic evaluation (see Chapter 2, as well as Sugden and Williams 1978; Culyer 1989).

Characteristic findings

In this section we will summarize the large empirical literature on revealed and expressed preferences.

Revealed preference findings

A review by de Blaeij et al. (2003) included only studies based on revealed preference. All studies utilized data related to road safety, either through the purchase of safer vehicles, related safety equipment or driving speeds. Monetary estimates were converted to US dollars by the authors according to purchasing power parity and an inflation adjustment was made to convert values into constant US dollars (in thousands). Dropping one outlier at each end, the estimates of VSL reported in this review range from approximately $3.0 million to $9.6 million, with most clustered at the low end. A review by Blomquist (2004) encompassed a few studies not included in de Blaeij et al. (2003), as well as two on non-automobile-related behaviour. Leaving aside motorcyclists, the range of VSL for adults is $5.6–14.4 million, with no particular bias toward either end. This review suggests a higher VSL than that found in de Blaeij et al. (2003).

Labour-market studies on VSL have been comprehensively summarized in Viscusi and Aldy (2003). Table 5.1 presents the majority of studies they cite that estimate a VSL using US labour-market data. We have excluded studies employing occupational and locational measures of risk, since these are less accurate than industrial attribution. The table indicates which studies employed a variable for non-fatal risk (failure to do so can result in the overestimation of wage compensation for fatal risk).

It is difficult to spot trends in the data. There is no overall tendency for later studies to generate higher VSLs than earlier ones, nor does the inclusion of a variable for non-fatal risk or differences in average income have the predicted effects. Heterogeneity in the estimates is driven primarily by the choice of samples, the use of different sources for measures of risk, and the choice of specification. It should be noted that, where researchers tried multiple specifications, Viscusi and Aldy selected those which, in their view, produced results most supportive of compensating differentials theory.

Table 5.2 presents the summary of non-US labour-market studies of fatal risk from Viscusi and Aldy (2003). The range is even greater for these studies, which employed a much wider variety of risk measures. In particular, there is only the slightest relationship between average worker income and average VSL.

Viscusi and Aldy also summarized 39 studies of non-fatal injury risk in the US. There is little value in reproducing this list, since the type and severity of injury differs from study to study and, since many of them did not control for income replacement by workers' compensation. Nearly all report statistically significant coefficients on risk, with the value of an injury lying primarily within the range of $20,000–120,000.

There has yet to be an exploration of injury-reporting bias in this literature. In most countries, data on fatal and non-fatal injuries are collected from employers, who have an incentive to under-report. This presumably plays a larger role in non-fatal than fatal injuries and there is evidence suggesting that under-reporting is most severe among small firms (Dorman 2000). If this is true, there would be a spurious size–risk relationship across firms and this would interact with the known size–wage relationship to generate spuriously positive coefficients on risk in wage equations. This would be a particular problem for studies that failed to control for firm size, which is to say nearly all of them.

Early labour-market studies of the VSL tended to give lower estimates than later ones, since they failed to account for the fact that wealthy people tend to choose safer jobs, an important endogeneity issue that well-designed studies can address by using simultaneous equation regression modelling (Jones-Lee 1989; Beattie et al. 1998a).

Table 5.1 Estimates of VSL from US labour-market data*.

Author	Non-fatal risk variable	Sample income mean	VSL in millions of $US 1,000
Smith (1974)	Yes	$29,029	18.4
Smith (1976)	Yes	$31,027	11.8
Viscusi (1978, 1979)	Yes	$31,842	10.6
Viscusi (1981)	Yes	$22,618	16.6
Olson (1981)	Yes	$36,151	13.4
Butler (1983)	No	$22,713	2.6
Dorsey and Walzer (1983)	Yes	$21,636	23.6, 24.6
Leigh and Folsom (1984)	Yes	$29,038 and $36,946	20.2–26.6
Smith and Gilbert (1984, 1985)	No		1.8
Dillingham and Smith (1984)	Yes	$29,707	8.2–16.6
Dillingham (1985)	No	$26,781	2.4, 6.4–13.6
Leigh (1987)	No		26.6
Moore and Viscusi (1988a)	No	$24,931	6.4, 18.8
Moore and Viscusi (1988b)	No	$31,092	19.4
Garen (1988)	Yes	$29,865	34.6
Viscusi and Moore (1989)	No	$24,611	20
Herzog and Schlottman (1990)	No	$48,364	23.4
Moore and Viscusi (1990a)	No	$24,611	41.6
Moore and Viscusi (1990b)	Yes	$24,611	41.6
Kniesner and Leeth (1991)	Yes	$33,627	1.4
Gegax et al. (1991)	No	$41,391	4.2
Leigh (1991)	No	$32,961	14.2–30.6
Berger and Gabriel (1991)	No	$46,865 and $48,029	17.2, 21.8
Leigh (1995)	No	$29,587	16.2–33.6
Dorman and Hagstrom (1998)	Yes	$32,243	17.4–40.6
Lott and Manning (2000)	No	$30,245	3, 6

* Source: Viscusi and Aldy (2003).

Table 5.2 Estimates of VSL from non-US labour-market data*.

Author	Country	Non-fatal risk variable	Mean sample income	VSL in millions of $US 1,000
Marin and Psacharopoulos (1982)	UK	No	$14,472	8.4
Weiss et al. (1986)	Austria	Yes	$12,011	7.8, 13
Meng (1989)	Canada	No	$43,840	7.8–9.4
Meng and Smith (1990)	Canada	No	$29,646	13–20.6
Kniesner and Leeth (1991)	Japan	Yes	$44,863	19.4
Kniesner and Leeth (1991)	Australia	Yes	$23,307	8.4
Cousineau et al. (1992)	Canada	Yes	$29,665	9.2
Martinello and Meng (1992)	Canada	Yes	$25,387	4.4–13.6
Kim and Fishback (1993)	South Korea	Yes	$8,125	1.6
Siebert and Wei (1994)	UK	Yes	$12,810	18.8–23
Lanoie et al. (1995)	Canada	Yes	$40,739	39.2–43.4
Sandy and Elliott (1996)	UK	No	$16,143	10.4–138.8
Shanmugam (1996/7)	India	No	$778	2.4, 3
Liu et al. (1997)	Taiwan	No	$5,007–6,088	0.4–1.8
Miller et al. (1997)	Australia	No	$27,177	2.6–38.2
Siebert and Wei (1998)	Hong Kong	No	$11,668	3.4
Liu and Hammitt (1999)	Taiwan	Yes	$18,483	1.4
Meng and Smith (1999)	Canada	Yes	$19,962	10.2–10.6
Arabsheibani and Marin (2000)	UK	Yes	$20,163	39.8
Shanmugam (2000)	India	Yes	$778	2, 2.8
Baranzini and Ferro Luzzi (2001)	Switzerland	No	$47,400	12.6, 17.2
Sandy et al. (2001)	UK	No	$16,143	11.4, 148.2
Shanmugam (2001)	India	Yes	$778	8.2

*Source: Viscusi and Aldy (2003).

Overall, the aspect of revealed preference analysis that causes the most difficulty is the tendency for different social groups to be assigned different values of life and health. Straightforward interpretations of VSL as valid measurements of intangible value are vexed by disturbing group-specific patterns in the empirical literature; selective use of these results, on the other hand, requires justifications that undermine the case for revealed preference analysis in the labour market altogether. This is most clearly seen in the union/non-union distinction, but applies to race and perhaps income as well.

A final concern that emerges is publication bias. Most researchers in the revealed preference field believe that properly conducted studies will find statistically significant values for life and health that roughly correspond to those already reported. Any paper submitted for publication would have to explain and validate non-conforming outcomes in ways not required for corroborative results. As a result, the sample of published papers, and the sub-sample of results that appears in influential literature reviews, is unlikely to be representative of the full breadth of research.

Expressed preference findings

The largest contingent valuation (CV) studies with nationally representative samples have been on road safety. There have been several in OECD countries, with largely similar results, and results that are also similar to those in well-designed revealed preference studies (Beattie *et al.* 1998a).

CV estimates of the VSL, however, vary considerably, with 700-fold variation between the highest and lowest estimates (Beattie *et al.* 1998a). Covey *et al.* (1995) estimated the value of a life from preventing food poisoning at £48,840,000 in 1995 prices, whereas Acton (1976) estimated the value of a life from preventing heart attacks at £69,800 in 1974 prices. One of the main drivers of this variation is the size of the risk reduction. Smaller risk reductions yield larger VSL. Covey *et al.* (1995) used an exceptionally small reduction in risk of death of 1.67 in 10 million, whereas Acton (1976) used an exceptionally large risk reduction of two in 1000. This phenomenon has been linked to a serious bias in CV, an under-sensitivity of WTA/WTP responses to the magnitude of risk reduction. Well-conducted experimental studies have found this bias to be particularly serious in relation to small health risks of the kind used in CV studies of the VSL (Beattie *et al.* 1998b).

Other drivers include the reference point (WTP for risk reduction yields lower values than WTA for risk increases), the sequencing of questions, the population subgroup (in particular their wealth and age), the hazard context (e.g., how voluntary the risk is), and the time horizon (e.g., whether reductions in current health risks from classic OHS programmes are valued more highly than equivalent reductions in future risks from disease management or health promotion programmes).

Studies that directly compare familiar hazard contexts, such as road safety, rail safety, food safety and air pollution, using CV techniques have generally found small variations in relative VSL of around ±50%. Jones-Lee *et al.* (1995) found a premium of 51% for underground fatalities relative to road accident fatalities. Cookson (2000) found variation of ±50% between six different contexts, with similar values for road, rail, and food safety, the value for air pollution about 50% higher, and the value for birth control pills and medical radiation about 50% lower. The main factor underlying such variations appears to be how voluntary the risk is perceived to be.

Anomalies in expressed preference studies

Systematic and persistent anomalies have been documented in expressed preference studies, both in the VSL and the wider economic literature on CV of non-market goods (Beattie *et al.* 1998a,b; Dubourg *et al.* 1997).

Some of the well-documented anomalies are: 1) protest zero responses (some individuals are unwilling to provide a valuation, as distinct from individuals with a zero valuation); 2) right skewness of responses (which has given rise to the use of median, rather than mean response); 3) undersensitivity to the magnitude of risk reduction (known variously as the embedding effect, part-whole bias, and scope/scale effects); and 4) oversensitivity to theoretically irrelevant cues (e.g., cost, baseline risk, payment card starting points and ranges, and the order in which items are valued). These anomalies are consistent with a substantial body of evidence from psychology and experimental economics, which suggests that individual preferences often do not conform to the economic model of rational choice (Loomes 1999). Anomalies are perhaps particularly striking with non-market goods that involve unfamiliar outcomes, small probabilities, and long time horizons. However, they have also been documented in relation to familiar household goods sold in the market place, such as mugs and chocolate bars.

One response to such anomalies is to improve survey design (Carson and Mitchell 1995). However, the pervasive nature of these anomalies suggests that they may reflect fundamental features of individuals' psychology and preference, and are not only due to shortcomings in survey design. A second is to use deliberative opinion polling techniques that allow respondents opportunities for deliberation and reflection, together with a battery of inconsistency checks, opportunities to revise preferences in the light of feedback, and qualitative research to investigate people's reasons for their responses in order to uncover more considered preferences. A third is to re-design value elicitation survey instruments so as to place less of a cognitive burden on the respondent and gain a better focus on the central valuation issues at hand. For example, questions about health-health trade-offs may be easier for respondents to tackle than CV questions about wealth-health trade-offs. A combination of all three responses may also be appropriate.

Using off-the-shelf value of safety estimates in practice

Two main practical questions face the researcher wishing to incorporate a monetary value of life or injury into an applied economic evaluation of an OHS intervention:

1) What base case and range of values should be selected from the thousands of off-the-shelf values reported?

2) Once the human outcomes of injury and disease have been valued in monetary terms, should the researcher add in financial outcomes such as loss of earnings or is this double counting?

There is no general algorithm for selecting the most appropriate base case monetary value of life or injury for economic evaluation. In general, the appropriate base case value will depend on the policy context (e.g., the cause of risk and the characteristics of those at risk). It is known, for example, that how voluntary the physical risk is typically contributes up to three-fold variation in the VSL. Other factors may contribute even larger variations. There can thus be a trade-off between the policy relevance of the study and its scientific quality. Whatever the base case, given the high degree of variability in estimates and the serious methodological concerns about methods, it is wise to conduct sensitivity analyses. Sensible ranges of estimates for sensitivity analysis might include: 1) the typical range suggested by current reviews of revealed preference studies; 2) the typical range suggested by current reviews of expressed preference studies; and 3) the typical range currently used by other relevant national or international decision-making bodies. For example, a recent review of revealed preference estimates of the value of preventing a single fatality from US labour-market studies suggested a reasonable range of $4–9 million in 2004 prices (Viscusi and Aldy 2005). Below we give examples of estimates used by two major UK government bodies.

It is also hard to provide definitive practical guidance on the question of double counting human and financial outcomes. A sensible guiding principle is that a worker's lost earnings should either be counted as a human outcome (i.e., as part of individual WTP for safety) or as a financial outcome (i.e., as part of lost output), but not both. An analyst may wish to separate the value a worker attaches to her/his own earnings (a human outcome) from the worker's net contribution to national output (a financial outcome). This is not entirely satisfactory from a conceptual point of view since a worker's net contribution to national output ultimately also has human consequences in terms of the value other individuals place on the worker's own consumption. Essentially, output and consumption are two sides of the same coin and each is subject to measurement error. Empirically, it is difficult to disentangle the component of individual WTP for safety attributable to loss of livelihood from components attributable to other factors, such as the loss of life, and the pain and suffering of relatives and friends.

UK Department for Transport values for preventing fatalities and injuries

The UK Department for Transport most recently reported an average value for preventing a single fatal casualty of £1,428,180 in 2005 prices (Department for Transport 2007). This is made up of three components: 1) lost output of £490,960, representing the present value of expected loss of earnings plus employer non-wage payments such as pension contributions; 2) medical and ambulance costs of £840; and 3) human costs of £936,380, representing the pain and suffering and loss of enjoyment of life. The third element is derived from a series of large national expressed preference studies conducted in the late 1990s and is adjusted for inflation. It is based on the CV approach (Jones-Lee *et al.* 1995; Carthy *et al.* 1999), minus an estimate of lost lifetime consumption. The corresponding value for preventing a serious injury is £160,480 (including human costs of £130,110) and for preventing a slight injury is £12,370 (including human costs of £9,530).

The NICE value of a Quality-Adjusted Life-Year (QALY)

The UK National Institute for Health and Clinical Excellence (NICE) draws heavily on economic techniques to guide the National Health Service (NHS) in making choices about health care technologies. It values health improvements using a Quality-Adjusted Life-Year (QALY) approach, rather than the WTP approach. NICE's own official estimate of the maximum monetary value of a marginal QALY lies between £25,000 and £35,000 (Rawlins and Culyer 2004). One analysis of historical decisions made by NICE suggests that the monetary value actually adopted is somewhat higher, at around £30,000 to £45,000 in 2005 prices (Parkin and Devlin 2006). The QALY threshold adopted by NICE does not represent the sum of individual willingness to pay for reductions in health risk. Rather, it represents NICE's estimate of the amount of money the UK National Health Service typically has available to spend at the margin to improve health (i.e., to purchase the corresponding number of QALYs).

It is possible to convert monetary VSL into monetary values for a QALY (and vice versa), by making various modelling assumptions about the remaining length and quality of life of the relevant at-risk population (Hirth *et al.* 2000; Mason *et al.* 2006). The most recent and sophisticated exercise of this kind was based on the 2003 UK Department for Transport's marginal value for preventing a fatality of £1,311,490 (i.e., the full 2003 value less medical and ambulance costs). This generated values for a QALY ranging from £6,000 to £63,000 with a preferred range from £45,000 to £60,000. The threshold value of a QALY currently adopted by NICE (i.e., ranging from £25,000 to £45,000) could thus be expected to translate into a VSL somewhat lower than the UK Department for Transport value.

One possible interpretation of this discrepancy is that the NICE value is too low and that the NHS budget should be expanded to allow government spending on health improvement in the health care field to match government spending on health improvement in the transport field. Another interpretation is that government spending on health improvement in the transport field is too high or that there are independent reasons for spending more on health improvements from investment in the transport field (e.g., because the health risks generally relate to younger individuals). A third is that the methodological challenges of valuing life and health are so great, and the theory and evidence used in the two different policy sectors are so different and so fraught with uncertainty and potential bias, that this apparent discrepancy is in fact remarkably small given the bounds of error that might reasonably be expected.

Methodological caveats and challenges

In conclusion, we emphasize some of the methodological challenges and caveats that beset this area, in the hope of encouraging further methodological work specifically related to the OHS arena.

First, although literature reviews often cite apparently narrow preferred ranges of values, the full range of values in the literature is much wider. Preferred ranges of values cited by reviews are always somewhat selective and, inevitably, those selections are based on the value judgments (not always openly stated) of the investigators.

Second, when interpreting the results of a particular valuation study, the devil is in the details. That is to say, the findings of both revealed and expressed preference studies are highly dependent, often in systematic ways, on the details of the study design and the methods of statistical analysis. The use of any particular value in practice should always be preceded by appropriately designed sensitivity analyses.

Third, much of the existing theoretical and empirical literature on valuing safety draws heavily on standard preference-based welfare economic theory. It would be helpful to have alternative approaches based on competing theories, for purposes of comparison and to test the sensitivity of the outcome to the choice of method.

Fourth, revealed preference analysis should ideally be accompanied by research indicating the degree to which risk perceptions of the target population are in accordance with objective measures of risk, to the extent that the latter can be determined. There is little merit in using subjective valuations that are based on factually objective error.

Fifth, given the serious methodological problems in setting an absolute monetary value using CV, an approach that employs relative valuation warrants further investigation and development. Such studies should ideally be accompanied by experimental checks on the internal consistency of responses, and by other efforts to identify and minimize bias, which might include qualitative research to identify the reasons underlying quantitative responses and providing opportunities for respondents to arrive at more considered responses.

Sixth, more attention should be given to the problem of group-specific and context-specific VSL. The idea that there should be a single, universally applicable monetary VSL for use in all settings is not supported by economic theory or evidence. The appropriate value is likely to depend upon the characteristics of the population group and the nature of the hazard. The size of these differences in practice and the extent to which they should be recognized and incorporated into policy analysis, are open questions.

Finally, we return to the issue of whether or not human as opposed to financial outcomes need to be quantified in monetary terms. An alternative approach would be to measure and report the full range of human outcomes in non-monetary units (e.g., lives saved, injuries and diseases of different kinds avoided, QALYs gained) and possibly break them down by different population groups, without attempting to value them in monetary terms or reduce them to a single figure representing the overall benefit. This alternative approach is sometimes known as cost–consequence analysis (Drummond et al. 2005). The choice of approach raises important philosophical issues about the role of economic evidence in the policy decision-making process. Cost–consequence analysis requires decision makers to use their own judgment and discretion in weighing the value of the different human outcomes, whereas CBA performs that valuation task for them. Ultimately, this methodological choice is as much a political question as a technical one about how much discretion should be left to the decision-making authority.

Appendix: empirical methodology

There are two general strategies for estimating trade-offs between income and safety: revealed and expressed preferences. Revealed preference techniques record actual market behaviour in the presence of differing levels of risk and attempt to isolate the role that risk plays in altering prices. Expressed preference methods employ questionnaires to directly ask individuals how much they might pay or accept for a given change in risk.

Revealed preference approaches

Using this approach, researchers utilize demand or supply data to estimate a relationship between changes in risk and offsetting monetary flows. By far the largest number of studies of VSL examines the labour market. In nearly every instance researchers employ the regression equation:

$$\ln(\text{wage}) = \text{constant} + \beta_1 \times \text{risk} + \beta_2 \times x_1 + \beta_3 \times x_2 + \dots + \varepsilon \qquad [1]$$

Here, the natural logarithm of the wage is employed, since the principle of diminishing marginal utility of income implies that equal percentage changes in income are more likely to correspond to equal increments of utility than equal absolute changes in income. In this specification β_1 is the coefficient on the risk variable, the x's are various worker characteristics that might affect earnings, each with its own coefficient, and ε is an error term. Samples are usually drawn from groups of workers concentrated in relatively more hazardous occupations; that is, workers from manufacturing, construction and extractive industries are likely to be over sampled relative to the population as a whole.

Let us first consider the theory behind this equation. The jobs that pay the highest wages (e.g., chemical engineering) are also likely to be relatively safe, while those that are the riskiest (e.g., meat cutting) pay less. Presumably, the workers with the best jobs have qualifications that give them access to the higher rungs of the labour market, whereas those whose skills are less in demand must choose between less desirable options. Thus, controlling for a range of worker characteristics is supposed to isolate the wage–risk relationship to more narrowly circumscribed market positions. If this statistical strategy is successful, the coefficient on risk would measure the trade-off between jobs that compete for identically qualified workers. This model would be much more likely to exhibit wage-compensation-for-risk results than a model which failed to distinguish between highly qualified and less qualified workers. Also, note that only the job risk and the worker's characteristics are incorporated. This implies that other aspects of the employer or industry play no role in wage determination.

Several issues have emerged in the econometric practice of calculating VSL:

1) In principle, workers face multiple risks on the job and each has the potential to make its own contribution to wage determination. Very simply, one could sort them into fatal and non-fatal risks; this would yield two risk variables, $risk_f$ and $risk_{nf}$, and two coefficients, β_f and β_{nf}. In practice, however, most analysts include only one such variable, usually fatal risk. Assuming that fatal and non-fatal risks are correlated, this will have the effect of artificially inflating the estimate of β_f from which VSL calculations are drawn.

2) There is likely to be significant error in observations of risk at the individual level. We simply do not have data that tell us how much risk each worker faces. Consequently, the usual approach is to assign to each worker the average risk factor for her/his industry, occupation or industry/occupation cell. Because the error in this procedure is random, it reduces the potential magnitude and significance of the estimates. Moreover, by creating a variable risk with fewer true observations than the other variables in the equation, it alters the method by which statistical significance should be calculated. The antidote involves an application of the technique of clustering, but in practice it is rarely employed.

3) Conventional economic theory holds that wages are determined primarily by the worker's productivity characteristics, but available observations on x are not likely to capture them fully. This will bias estimates of the risk coefficient in ways that are unpredictable *a priori*.

4) Non-fatal risks are costly to workers in part due to their monetary effects, but some of these are defrayed by workers' compensation. In many jurisdictions benefits and coverage varies. In principle, whenever $risk_{nf}$ is employed, a variable that estimates workers' compensation coverage should be included as well.

5) For utility purposes, workers may be assumed to care only about their after-tax income, but data sets used by researchers often report only pre-tax income. In that case, adjustments should be made based on marginal tax rates applicable to each individual.

6) Many of the x variables describe categorical differences between workers, such as age, race, sex and union membership. The specification presented in [1] implicitly assumes that the coefficients on all independent variables are the same across these categories, but this may be wrong. For instance, it is not clear that experience, a standard x variable, should play the same

role in wage determination for men and women, or for whites and visible minorities. Ideally, each category should be estimated separately, although the data sets are not always large enough to permit this, particularly in light of the small sample error that would arise in particular industry/occupation cells. There may not be enough black workers, for instance, in each cell, even in the entire population, to generate a reliable observation on their level of risk or to reliably estimate its coefficient.

7) A different approach to age is to translate fatal risk into expected number of years lost, a quantity that falls with the worker's age and the extent of latency (if the risk is caused by a disease). In principle, this should yield a value per statistical life-year across individuals, although this may be age-related, as well as a consequence of either changing preferences or life-cycle income effects. For instance, young workers may be less risk-averse than older ones; also, if workers save income for retirement, they may attach more value to their retirement years than their working years.

8) A more recent concern is that workers may vary not only by productivity and risk preferences, but also by capacity for self-protection in dangerous jobs (Shogren and Stamland 2002). If this is the case, the error stemming from assigning average group risk to individuals within that group (see 2 above) will not be random, since safer workers will presumably require less wage compensation. This exacerbates the problem of measurement error on risk.

9) In most instances, researchers include only individual-level variables in x. This is in accordance with conventional economic theory, which holds that workers of equal productivity should receive equal utility packages in employment—the law of one price. Nevertheless, there is widespread evidence that employer characteristics play an important role in wage determination as well. This has been demonstrated in the inter-industry wage differential literature, where it has been shown that persistent wage premia attach to particular industries, even across disparate occupations such as secretaries and machine operators. Economists who have studied this phenomenon are likely to attribute it to rent-sharing: firms in some industries are able to make above-average profits, and they are under pressure from their workforce to share some of this in the form of above-average wages. To the extent that this is the case, estimates of wage compensation for risk will be biased if they fail to include variables that capture these employer- and industry-level effects. The simplest form that this can take is industry dummies, but labour-market research would endorse other variables as well, such as firm size, the firm's capital–labour

ratio and union density and gender composition at the industry level (Dorman and Hagstrom 1998).

From the standpoint of OHS policy, one irony implicit in the wage compensation literature is this: researchers are estimating VSLs on the basis of the assumption that all risk is fully compensated, yet these same values are often proposed as benchmarks to be used for evaluating public policies whose rationale depends on the failure of wage compensation.

Expressed preference approaches

The expressed preference approach that is most closely wedded to standard welfare economic theory is the CV approach. This focuses on hypothetical wealth–health trade-offs made by individuals (or households) between their own wealth, and specified risks to their own life and health. In essence, it asks individuals how much they are willing to pay for a specified risk reduction (or, less often, how much they are willing to accept for a specified increase in risk). Unfortunately, at least when applied to the relatively small changes in individual health risk delivered by most health and safety interventions, this approach runs into some serious biases and methodological challenges (Beattie *et al.* 1998a,b).

As a result, investigators have turned to alternative relative valuation approaches that ask respondents to make hypothetical trade-offs that are easier for respondents to handle from a cognitive point of view. These approaches may be somewhat less firmly grounded in standard welfare economic theory, but the advantage is that they place less cognitive strain on respondents and thus help to reduce some of the more serious biases and anomalies that have afflicted the standard CV approach.

One such approach is the chained CV/SG approach, which breaks the CV valuation task down into more manageable steps (Carthy *et al.* 1999). The first step involves standard CV questions involving trade-offs between wealth and a non-fatal injury, typically, both a question about WTP to be cured of the non-fatal injury and a question about WTA to remain injured. The second step is to ask a standard gamble (SG) question involving trade-offs between the certainty of a non-fatal injury and a risk of death. In this question, the respondents are asked to imagine a treatment for the non-fatal injury that carries a small risk of immediate death. They are then essentially asked what risk of immediate death they would accept in order to be cured of the non-fatal injury, thus giving a non-monetary, relative value of dying compared with the non-fatal injury. The monetary value of a non-fatal injury from the first step can then be chained to the relative value of dying compared with the non-fatal injury, to yield a monetary value of dying. This is the approach that has been adopted as the basis for the value for preventing a fatality currently used by the UK Department for Transport (Carthy *et al.* 1999; Department for Transport 2007).

More generally, the relative valuation (or relativities approach) focuses on valuation tasks that ask respondents to compare one health risk against another, for example, fatal versus non-fatal injury, different types of non-fatal injury, and different types of risk in different contexts. This allows one to develop a system of relative valuations for different health risks. In principle, this entire system of relative values can then be converted into a system of monetary values by attaching a monetary value to just one of the health risks, rather like hanging the system on a single monetary peg. Although developed in other policy sectors, one preliminary study suggests that this relativities approach may be a fruitful avenue to pursue in the OHS field (Karnon *et al.* 2005).

Relative valuation questions may involve risks to the individual's own health, as in the SG approach described above and as in the time-trade-off approach that involves trade-offs between length of time spent in different health states. Alternatively, relative valuation may involve risks to population health. For example, the person trade-off value elicitation technique asks individuals to make trade-offs between numbers of lives saved (or injuries prevented) from different policy interventions. This involves an important change of perspective from that of consumer (i.e., thinking about risks to one's own life and health) to that of citizen (i.e., thinking about risks to other people's life and health). It is a further departure from standard welfare economic theory, which adopts the consumer perspective.

These and other relative valuation techniques allow the investigator to establish relativities between values for preventing fatality and values for preventing non-fatal injury (e.g., see Jones-Lee *et al.* 1995), between values for different hazard contexts (e.g., see Jones-Lee and Loomes 1995) and, also, in principle, between different population subgroups. These relative values can then be converted into absolute monetary values by using one or more standard peg monetary values.

This chapter is an adapted version of Lessons from the literature on valuing reductions in physical risk, *Institute for Work & Health, Toronto, Working Paper #342, and has been reproduced with permission from the Institute of Work & Health.*

Chapter 6

The institutional and regulatory settings for occupational health and safety: an international survey

Ulrike Hotopp, John Mendeloff,
Sandra Sinclair, Emile Tompa,
Birgit Koeper, and Alan Clayton

Introduction

This chapter presents a survey of the institutional and regulatory context of occupational health and safety (OHS) systems in several jurisdictions. The intent of the survey is to provide readers with a sense of how the OHS context can vary from one jurisdiction to another and, hence, offer an appreciation of how different systems can affect workplace parties and other stakeholders in different ways. Key factors to keep in mind are the behavioural incentives created by a system, as well as its impact on outcomes, and the distribution of costs and consequences. These factors must be borne in mind when designing a study (some effects may be of more consequence in some jurisdictions than others), when comparing the results of evaluations done in different jurisdictions, or when assessing the implications of a study done in one jurisdiction for another. There is a significant diversity of policy environments even amongst jurisdictions having close geographical and cultural proximity. Given the importance of system incentives, it is good practice in the reporting of study results to clearly outline the OHS context in which the intervention was undertaken, and to highlight those aspects most relevant to behaviour, outcomes, and the distribution of costs and consequences in the jurisdiction(s) in question.

The survey is necessarily selective, providing broad summaries of the six systems. Each summary gives an overview:

- how disability insurance, health care services for occupational injury and disease, and OHS systems are organized;

- identifies the key stakeholders and institutional players;
- outlines the financing and delivery of benefits and services.

The summaries emphasize key characteristics to help readers appreciate the policy environments in which stakeholders (employers, labour unions, workers, governments, health care providers, and insurers) operate.

United States

Overview

Workers' compensation programmes in the United States are, with a few exceptions, legislated by state governments. Most were established around the time of World War I and embody the no-fault principle, which prohibits lawsuits against a worker's employer. Currently, about 96% of wage and salary workers are covered by workers' compensation. In all but four states, private insurance firms compete to provide the bulk of the coverage. The four states have an exclusive state fund for workers' compensation insurance, although three of these allow self-insurance. Twenty-one other states also have a competitive public insurer, which often provides coverage of last resort. In 2005, 56% of the $89 billion collected for insurance was received by private insurers, 21% by state funds, 18% by self-insured firms (primarily large firms), and 5% by federal government programmes. On the benefit side, in 2002, 11% of the payments were paid for permanent total disabilities and fatalities, 69% for permanent partial disabilities, and 20% for temporary total disabilities.

Workers' compensation insurers typically modify the premiums of employers for those risks whose experience provides an actuarial basis for prediction. States vary in the extent to which they impose ceilings or floors on premium modifications, although most rely on a similar formula, which considers the last three years of losses, weighting more recent experience more heavily. The size of losses for individual claims is generally capped at about $5,000, thus limiting the weight of injury severity relative to frequency.

In 1970, insurance premiums were 1.11% of covered payroll. That percentage increased to 1.96% by 1980, largely as a result of benefit increases. Some of the increases were spurred by recommendations of the National Commission on State Workmen's Compensation in 1971. From 1987 through 1994, insurance premiums exceeded 2% of covered payrolls, and then decreased to a low of 1.32% in 2000. The decrease was driven largely by a decline in claims, particularly lost-time claims. From 2003 to 2005, employer costs as a percentage of payroll remained between 1.7 and 1.75%. These national figures can obscure state level developments. For example, benefits paid to injured workers in California increased by 66% from 1999 to 2003, while they increased by only 14% in the rest of the nation.

Businesses and state officials frequently claim that high workers' compensation costs drive existing firms away from their state and deter new ones from entering. The declining membership and political strength of labour unions during the last two decades has weakened the demand for expanded benefits. Most public discussions about workers' compensation treat the reduction in workers' compensation costs as a desirable objective, without considering how costs would be reduced, and what the implication of such reductions would be. Most of the cost-cutting measures focus less on the size of the indemnity benefits than on reducing incentives to file claims, and on restricting high-cost and long-duration medical treatments.

Workers' compensation insurance

Workers' compensation insurance covers health care expenses and provides wage replacement benefits for work disability associated with occupational injury and disease. Payments for health care expenses, which were only one-third of total benefits in 1970, now total roughly 50% of expenditures, a growth largely reflecting the overall national rise in health care spending. Each state currently has rules regarding health care coverage under workers' compensation, but until the 1990s, it was largely free from the restrictions being imposed on health care coverage paid for from other sources, both private and public. The rising share and absolute volume of health care expenses in workers' compensation has generated great interest in setting limits on treatments, choice of provider, and prices. The quality of the health care treatment provided to injured workers is also beginning to emerge as a topic of discussion.

The adequacy and equity of lost-wage replacement by workers' compensation is a subject of continuing controversy. The evidence that workers are not fully compensated is strong, but confronts concerns about both moral hazard and jurisdictional competition. These concerns are unusually strong in the US—the former concern probably because of cultural, ethnic, and racial diversity, and the latter because of the number of jurisdictions, and relatively limited federal government control. Compensation of occupational diseases, especially those with long latency periods, has been particularly poor. For example, byssinosis was unacknowledged in the US as an occupational disease, even while it was being compensated in Great Britain. Although disease claims have more recently been facilitated, the uncompensated burden remains high. For example, in most Canadian provinces cases of asbestos-related disease in recent years comprise about 20% of compensated fatalities, a much larger share than in the United States.

Other sources of disability compensation

As noted above, workers' compensation legislation does not allow lawsuits against an injured worker's employer. However, lawsuits against third parties who supply materials and equipment have been noteworthy. Those spawned by asbestos-related disease are by far the most common. Although the legal standard for assessing liability has, in theory, changed from negligence to strict liability, in practice it is often hard to distinguish between the two. The single most important element in many toxic chemical cases has been a 'failure to warn.' As a result, chemical producers have supported the efforts of the Occupational Safety and Health Administration (OSHA), as well as private initiatives, to raise awareness of hazards and encourage good practice.

Regarding alternative compensation systems coverage, an injured worker often has a choice of the compensation system from which to draw benefits. For example, although employment-based health insurance is not provided by all employers and has become less common than it was, the health care coverage for most workers is still of this type. Similarly, many employers provide paid sick leave regardless of cause. If an employer's workers' compensation premiums are more sensitive to occupational injury and disease expenses than to other mechanisms, there is an incentive for the firm to shift expenses to the other third-party payers.

The federal Social Security Disability Insurance (SSDI) programme is the largest payer of disability benefits. In 2005, it supported 6.8 million disabled workers and 1.8 million of their dependents. SSDI is paid for through payroll taxes and is limited to individuals who are permanently disabled. About 1.4 million workers on SSDI received benefits from workers' compensation or some other public disability programme. SSDI rules require that the benefits from different programmes be coordinated such that an injured worker does not receive more than 80% of pre-injury earnings. In the 1970s, workers' compensation wage-replacement benefits were lower than SSDI benefits, but surpassed them by 1983 and remained higher until 1994. Since 1995, workers' compensation benefits have, once again, become lower. In fact, by 2005 SSDI benefits were about 80% higher than workers' compensation benefits. It appears that systems other than workers' compensation are covering some of the cost of occupational injuries and diseases, although workers' compensation may be paying for some non-occupational injuries and diseases. These cross-subsidies, along with the fact that payments to injured workers can vary based on where the exposure occurred (e.g., whether a slip and fall occurred at work, at home, or at the department store), provide support for a universal, no-fault system for all injuries, diseases and disabilities.

However, labour unions have generally not endorsed the idea of a universal programme, and both trial lawyers and workers' compensation officials strongly oppose it.

Prevention incentives

Along with other goals like compensation and restorative justice, prevention is an important goal of the workers' compensation system. The provision of insurance pools risks and can weaken prevention incentives. The experience rating of premiums is a step towards restoring these incentives. In addition, insurers provide advice and incentives through other measures. Most states have laws requiring workers' compensation insurers to provide loss control services to their customers. However, these measures can encourage firms to dispute legitimate claims, as well as investing in prevention.

OSHA is the most visible public agency involved in prevention. OSHA came into existence through the Occupational Safety and Health Act, which was passed into legislation by a Democratic congress and a Republican president in 1970. Its creation primarily reflects organized labour's desire for a stronger federal presence in OHS. The Act reflected suspicion of bureaucratic timidity and the potential capture of the regulators by the regulated. To counter these, the Act included a number of mandates that the agency had to follow and gave it a strict timetable. The Act also empowered workers to some degree by requiring the agency to respond to requests for inspections, allow workers the opportunity to accompany inspectors, and post citations with abatement dates so that compliance could be monitored.

Most of the standards adopted by OSHA in 1971 had been developed by private standard-setting organizations. These organizations typically made decisions by consensus using a criterion of reasonableness. OSHA's standards included thousands of specific requirements. It soon became apparent that, despite the consensus approach by which the standards were developed, many firms did not fully comply and, in some cases, the rules were outdated. As a result, OSHA faced heavy criticism for its 'nitpicking.'

During the first two decades of OSHA's existence, almost all its health standards were challenged in court. Along with other US regulatory programmes, it faced increasing judicial demands to provide stronger evidence to justify its decisions. OSHA was required to assess whether compliance with each standard was feasible in every industrial category, and whether each addressed a significant risk. The latter task required quantitative risk assessment. The courts affirmed that OSHA did not need to establish health standards on the basis of cost–benefit analyses, but required the standards to be the most protective ones feasible. A statute mandating the lowest feasible level of exposure and a high burden of proof made it difficult for regulators to take moderate steps on the basis of limited evidence. Hence, few standards were adopted, but those that were tended to be relatively stringent.

Prior to the creation of OSHA, state enforcement had rarely relied on fines or prosecutions. Under OSHA, administrative fines are mandatory for serious violations. However, employers can appeal against citations and penalties, first to an independent Occupational Safety and Health Review Commission and then to the federal courts. OSHA penalties remained relatively low until the late 1980s, when it began introducing the first million dollar fines. About 40% of inspections lead to fines and the average fine is several thousand dollars.

The Occupational Safety and Health Act allows state governments to take responsibility for regulatory enforcement with the stipulation that the federal OSHA first determine that the state programme is at least as effective as the federal programme. Twenty-one states with about 40% of national employment have taken on the responsibility. Typically, they employ more compliance officers *per capita* and inspect a larger fraction of the firms in their states than the federal body does in states for which it has oversight. However, they levy fewer fines and penalties. About 80% of all inspections are in manufacturing and construction workplaces.

Overall, the average penalty per inspection is higher in the United States than in Canada or European jurisdictions, although the number of compliance officers and inspections is between one-third and one-tenth of these other jurisdictions. Regulation in the US has an element of toughness, but it is weakened by limited resources. The greater toughness entails more procedures and less flexibility.

Selected websites on the American OHS system

Center to Protect Worker Rights: www.cpwr.com
National Council on Compensation Insurance: www.ncci.com
RAND Center for Health and Safety in the Workplace: www.rand.org/multi/chsw
US Bureau of Labor Statistics: www.bls.gov
US National Institute for Occupational Safety and Health: www.cdc.gov/niosh
US Occupational Safety and Health Administration: www.osha.gov
Workers Compensation Research Institute: www.wcrinet.org

Canada

Overview

Canada is a highly decentralized federation made up of 10 provinces and three territories. The national government has jurisdiction over issues of national interest, such as the regulation of trade and commerce, postal services, defence, employment insurance, and administration of the territories. Provincial governments have jurisdiction over natural resources, the administration and delivery of health care services, municipal institutions, property and civil rights, education, labour legislation, social security, and the creation of local governments (municipal, metropolitan, or regional). Some responsibilities are shared by the two levels of government. These include agriculture, immigration, some aspects of natural resources, public pensions, public and environmental health, health promotion, and health care financing. With regard to the latter, legislation in 1957 established a national health care system in which the federal government provided transfer payments to the provinces to support the provision of universal health care services. The federal transfers were conditional: provincial health care services had to meet federally established standards, the key one being that residents of the provinces had to have access to medically necessary services without direct charge. Given that labour legislation and health care are provincial level jurisdictions, the OHS system (including regulation and insurance), and the health care system vary somewhat from province to province, though there are many common features.

OHS and workers' compensation insurance

In addition to employment standards legislation which establishes minimum requirements and obligations for employment relationships, there are two major responsibilities that fall on the OHS systems in provincial/territorial jurisdictions: OHS legislation and workers' compensation. Generally, OHS legislation sets out the rights and duties of all parties in the workplace. It aims to protect workers against health and safety hazards through procedures, education and training; inspection and monitoring; and the enforcement of the law in the absence of voluntary compliance. Workers' compensation legislation establishes the agency responsible for the delivery of workers' compensation programmes, and its responsibilities in the spheres of prevention, rehabilitation, and compensation.

The government department responsible for prevention varies across jurisdictions. In some, it is the ministry or Department of Labour. In others, it belongs to a workers' compensation board. In yet others, the responsibilities are shared between a ministry and a compensation agency. In British Columbia, Quebec, New Brunswick, and Prince Edward Island, the agency responsible for workers' compensation also has regulatory responsibility for the inspectorate and enforcement aspects of OHS. In most of the other jurisdictions the regulatory responsibility lies with a separate institution, either the provincial ministry of labour or a separate OHS commission.

Under their OHS acts, all Canadian provinces and territories fund and support health and safety education programmes, training, and research aimed at prevention. In the province of Ontario, for example, 12 industry-based, and two cross-sectoral health and safety associations provide prevention-focused training programmes and related products and services to the province's employers and workers.

In Canada there is a strong reliance on internal responsibility to promote prevention. It is founded on the principle that everyone in the workplace, both workers and employers, is responsible for safety. Legislation does not always impose or prescribe the specific steps required for compliance. Rather, joint health and safety committees, consisting of labour and management representatives, are the key administrative element through which the internal responsibility system is put into practice. In general, such committees are mandatory for workplaces with 20 or more employees. They have roles in the development of health and safety programmes, monitoring injury, disease and work hazards, resolving complaints and work refusals, and making recommendations to management.

Canadian workers' compensation systems are modelled on the Meredith principles dating back to 1914 and are similar to the earlier German model. Both are essentially exclusive remedy systems, i.e., there is no recourse to tort law. They operate on the principle of no fault, providing collective liability for employers and compulsory insurance coverage for workers, through publicly administered, not-for-profit, monopolistic insurance agencies. Workers' compensation is a social insurance mechanism established to protect workers from the physical and financial impact of injury and disease sustained in the course of employment. It also provides employers with protection from costly litigation. Under the authority of their respective ministries of labour, workers' compensation agencies function as administrators of the legislative act that binds them, the insurers, the adjudicating tribunals, and the providers (or at least the third-party payers) of medical and rehabilitative services.

While many programmatic variances exist regarding indemnity and other benefits, workers' compensation programmes across the country in general cover the costs of health care and other treatment, vocational rehabilitation expenses and lost earnings associated with occupational injury and disease. The four major forms of benefit include: wage replacement on a temporary basis until return to work, typically in the order of 70% of gross earnings or 90% of net earnings, subject to a maximum and minimum; permanent disability payments for workers with continuing residual impairment, typically for lost earnings, and, in some instances, for non-economic losses and forgone retirement savings; fatality or survivor benefits in cases where a worker dies from the occupational injury or disease; and health care and other medical rehabilitation services purchased from the universal coverage health care plans within each jurisdiction. Workers are free to choose their own health care provider within the provincial programme and all services prescribed by the attending physician for the occupational injury or disease are paid for by the insurer. Return-to-work and labour market re-entry programmes are provided for injured workers and survivors where necessary.

Workers' compensation covers between 65 and 100% of workers in Canada, with considerable variation across provincial/territorial jurisdictions. Coverage in terms of scope/type of injury/disease, while more consistent across the jurisdictions, is by no means comprehensive. Compensation for some conditions (chronic stress and repetitive strain injuries are two) may be restricted or precluded from coverage. The compensation system is financed by payroll taxes levied on employers that average about 3% of covered payroll, with some variation by industry, reflecting different risk and accident experiences. Virtually all jurisdictions have introduced financial incentives for firms through experience rating, which links the firm's premium rate to the cost of its actual claims experience.

Other sources of disability compensation

Work disability benefits are also available from other sources. A federally administered pension programme called the Canada Pension Plan (CPP) provides disability, pension and survivor benefits for all workers in nine of the ten provinces and the three territories. The province of Quebec has its own, parallel plan called the Quebec Pension Plan (QPP) with similar provision for all workers in Quebec. The CPP/QPP programmes are financed 50/50 by workers and employers through payroll contributions determined by a set fraction of insurable earnings, the latter being determined by the average industrial wage. Self-employed individuals pay 100% of the insurance premium. To be eligible for disability benefits, a claimant must have made contributions for a minimum number of years, and be wholly or substantially disabled (benefits are not provided for partial work disability). In most jurisdictions there is financial offset of benefits from workers' compensation if CPP/QPP benefits are received concurrently with workers' compensation benefits for an occupational injury or disease.

Some employers also provide wage-replacement benefits for general sickness absences and short- and long-term disability that is not compensable through workers' compensation. These programmes are not obligatory, consequently only some employers offer them. The formal burden of financing these disability benefits falls wholly or partially on the employer. Portions not falling on employers come from workers through payroll deductions. For some short- and long-term disability programmes, employers purchase insurance through private insurance carriers. In principle, a worker is not eligible for wage-replacement benefits from a private insurer if the absence is attributable to a compensable occupational injury or disease. A workers' compensation claim must be made for such conditions.

The federally administered Employment Insurance Program is another source of short-term benefits for individuals not able to continue their employment due to injury or disease. This is formally financed by workers' and employers (50/50) through payroll contributions determined by a set fraction of insurable earnings. To be eligible, a worker has to contribute for a minimum number of weeks.

Finally, the Social Security programme (a provincial level jurisdiction) also offers means-tested benefits for individuals unable to work due to disability. These benefits are financed from general taxes.

Health care financing and delivery

Health care administration and delivery is a provincial/territorial responsibility. Services are financed by both the federal government (through transfer payments to the provinces and territories) and the provincial/territories governments through general taxes. The delivery systems are private, and are mostly not-for-profit hospitals and physicians operating as sole proprietors. Physicians bill the provincial/territorial programmes for their services on a pre-negotiated fee schedule. For medically necessary health care needs that are not associated with a workers' compensation claim, residents access health care services primarily through their general practitioner. Services covered through the provincial/territorial health care plan focus on ambulatory and hospital-based diagnosis and treatment of acute and chronic diseases, and on rehabilitation. Home care and prescription drug coverage is limited.

As noted, workers' compensation agencies in each jurisdiction also draw extensively on the health care delivery system for services for workers with compensable injuries and diseases. Payment for these services is financed through premiums paid for by employers, rather than from general tax coffers, and rates may differ from those negotiated with providers by the province. In some cases, a premium is paid for expedited services. Given the parallel nature of the health care financing and delivery for compensable, occupational injuries, and diseases, health care in Canada can be considered multi-tiered.

Another tier is health care services for injuries associated with vehicle accidents, which are fully financed by motor vehicle insurance providers. In most provinces these providers are private, for-profit, businesses, although four provinces (British Columbia, Saskatchewan, Manitoba, and Quebec) have a public, not-for-profit motor vehicle insurance administered by the provincial government. In the first three, private insurers provide top-up insurance to enhance the basic coverage provided by the public insurance. In Quebec, expenses related to injury and mortality are covered by public insurance, while private insurers provide coverage for vehicle and property damage, as well as expenses associated with injuries arising from accidents outside the province.

Yet another tier of health care is that provided to members of the Canadian military. Its health care needs are delivered by a specialized, not-for-profit health care system funded by the federal government. Similarly, the federal government provides primary care services on First Nations reserves and in isolated areas where no provincial/territorial services are available.

Selected websites on the Canadian OHS system

Canadian Association of Workers' Compensation Boards: www.awcbc.org
Human Resources and Social Development Canada:
    www.hrsdc.gc.ca/en/lp/lo/fwcs/boards.shtml
Institute for Work & Health: www.iwh.on.ca
Institut de recherche Robert-Sauvé en santé et en sécurité du travail: www.irsst.qc.ca
Canada Pension Plan: www1.servicecanada.gc.ca/en/isp/cpp/cpptoc.shtml
Québec Pension Plan: www.rrq.gouv.qc.ca/en/programmes/regime_rentes
Health Canada: www.hc-sc.gc.ca/hcs-sss/index_e.html

United Kingdom

Overview

The UK is a constitutional monarchy, with a national parliament in London and three separate parliaments/assemblies, one in Edinburgh (for Scotland), another in Cardiff (for Wales), and a third in Belfast (for Northern Ireland). England has nine regions, but these do not have devolved powers comparable with the three separate parliaments/assemblies. Local government (local authorities or Local Councils in Northern Ireland) plays a role in the design of local policies, and in the enforcement of national legislation including health and safety. The policy areas devolved to Scotland, Wales, and Northern Ireland differ. While responsibility for the health system has been split between the administrations of Scotland, England, Wales, and Northern Ireland, both the welfare system and OHS remain reserved (non-devolved) matters for which the UK Parliament retains full control. The Department for Business, Enterprise, and Regulatory Reform is responsible for labour-market regulations. Within this general framework the UK national Parliament retains the power to legislate on any issue, devolved or not.

There are a number of social partners in the OHS system. Those representing employers include the Confederation of British Industry, the Institute of Directors, Federation of Small Businesses, Chemical Industries Association and Engineering Employers Federation. Trade unions representing workers include a number of individual unions representing various areas of work. Most unions are members of the Trades Union Congress in England, Scotland, and Wales, In addition, there are several professional organizations with particular interests in OHS, such as the Royal Institute of Chartered Surveyors (construction industry) and the Chartered Institute of Personnel Development (sickness absence and stress management). Other OHS organizations include the Institution of Occupational Safety and Health as well as the Royal Society for the Prevention of Accidents. Local authorities are represented by the Local Authorities Coordinators of Regulatory Services, the Local Government Association, and their Scottish, Northern Irish, and Welsh equivalents.

The OHS system

The Health and Safety Executive (HSE) is governed by the HSE Board, a group of up to 11 individuals who are non-executive directors of the HSE and the HSE's senior management team. Members of the HSE Board are appointed by the Secretary of State for Work and Pensions and represent employers, workers, local authorities, and the public interest. The senior management team consists of 13 civil servants including the HSE's Chief Executive Officer. This structure has replaced the former dual structure in which the Health and Safety Commission (HSC) guided policymaking and the HSE implemented HSC policies.

The new HSE's primary function is to develop policy to protect the health, safety, and welfare of people at work, and the public at large. It is independent and reflects the interests of the social partners and local government. OHS legislation is enforced by both HSE and local authorities, depending on the main activity carried out at a particular worksite. Locally enforced sectors include distribution, retail, office, leisure and catering industries.

The basis for most OHS law in the UK is the 1974 Health and Safety at Work Act. The underlying principle of the act is the assessment and reduction of risk. Those who create risks to workers and the general public are responsible for their protection. Employers are responsible for providing a safe work environment in co-operation with their workers. The act also extends to the self-employed. Regulations are laws, approved by parliament and are usually made under the Health and Safety at Work Act, following proposals from the HSE Board, including proposals based on EU directives. Approved Codes of Practice offer practical examples of good practice and give advice on how to comply with the law. Approved Codes of Practice have legal force. Inspectors enforce the OHS legislation. They offer advice, warn duty holders, where appropriate serve improvement and prohibition notices and can ultimately prosecute through the courts. The detailed steps differ in the devolved administrations.

OHS support services are provided by both the public and private sectors. The HSE publishes guidance on a range of OHS issues. Guidance can be specific to the OHS concerns of an industry or of a particular process used in a number of industries. The main purpose of guidance is to interpret regulations and give technical advice. There are two other public programmes, one recently begun in England and Wales, and one in Scotland. Workplace Health Connect is a pilot OHS support service that began in England and Wales in early spring 2006. This service is available on demand to small- and medium-sized employers of up to 250 workers. It provides a helpline offering advice, specific problem solving advice, and site visits from OHS specialists. Safe and Healthy Working is an OHS service for employers and workers in small- and medium-sized enterprises in Scotland. Its services include a free and confidential helpline, site visits from OHS specialists, and a website that provides advice and guidance. The Small Business Advisory Service in Northern Ireland advises small and emerging businesses on how to effectively manage health and safety of their workforce. In terms of private sector services, a large and competitive market has developed for the sale of OHS advice, assessments and support. Services are often tailored to fit the type and size of the business seeking OHS support. OHS services are also provided through intermediaries such as insurance companies, banks, trade associations and trade unions, either as part of an insurance policy or as benefit of membership.

Disability compensation programmes

The Department for Work and Pensions, created in 2001, is responsible for the social security system, including disability compensation, unemployment insurance, state pensions, and other benefit programmes. There are several programmes providing compensation to individuals with disabilities. We describe each of these below.

Wage and salaried workers (but not the self-employed) qualify for Industrial Injuries Disablement Benefits if they experience disability associated with an occupational injury or disease. In order to claim the benefits a worker must have been employed at the time of accident or exposure to the disease agent. The severity of disability is assessed by a general practitioner, who estimates a percentage of total bodily impairment. This percentage is used to determine the level of benefit received.

Workers who experience an occupational injury or disease are also entitled to benefits under the state social security system. The Industrial Injuries

Scheme provides preferential social security benefits for disability arising from occupational injury or disease.

All employers are required by law to purchase Employers Liability Compulsory Insurance to cover their civil liabilities. This insurance is provided by private insurance carriers, who also provide preventive services such as evaluating high-risk worksites. Employment Liability Compulsory Insurance insures employers against the costs of compensation for workers who experience an occupational injury or disease for which the employer is at fault. The insurance provides compensation to injured workers of the at-fault employer. Most claims are paid only after claimants are successful at winning their case in court.

Individuals unable to work due to a disability (not necessarily caused by work) may also be eligible for Incapacity Benefits. Claimants for these benefits require an assessment by a general practitioner, who may recommend further medical examination. Individuals receiving Industrial Injuries Disablement Benefits and Incapacity Benefits may also be entitled to increases in other benefits such as child tax credits, depending on the size of their family, and the value of other benefits and income received.

Individuals may also qualify for Disability Living Allowances if they are under the age of 65 at the time of claiming, and have a serious physical or mental disability such that they require assistance with self-care or have difficulty walking. Receipt of Disability Living Allowance is not dependent on an individual working and is generally not means tested. The programme has two parts: a care component and a mobility component. Each component is paid at a different rate according to the impact of the disability on self-care and mobility.

Health care financing and delivery

The National Health Service (NHS) is the primary provider of health care in the UK, though there is also a small private sector for health care. The NHS is funded through contributions paid for by employers and workers.

In England the Department of Health is responsible for policies regarding the provision of health care including the NHS, public and mental health issues, general social services, including community care and care for the elderly, support to UK health care and the pharmaceutical industry. The Department of Health sets standards and oversees their implementation. There are ten Strategic Health Authorities that are responsible for managing and setting the strategic direction of the NHS at the local level. They are the key link between the NHS and the Department of Health.

In Wales, the Welsh Department for Health and Social Services funds and sets the policy for health services. It works in partnership with NHS. Local health boards are responsible for determining the needs of their constituents and commissioning services from NHS to meet those needs.

In Scotland, the Scottish Executive Health Department is responsible for the development and implementation of health and community care policy. It works in partnership with NHS Scotland, which oversees the Scottish health service. The service consists of 14 territorial boards that plan and deliver all health care services in their area.

The Northern Irish Department of Health, Social Services and Public Safety delivers health and social care, public health and public safety including fire services. Four health and social services boards (agencies of the Department of Health), commission and purchase services in their area.

Selected websites on the OHS system in the United Kingdom

Health and Safety Executive: www.hse.gov.uk

Department of Health: www.dh.gov.uk

Safety and Health Working: www.dh.gov.uk/en/Aboutus/HowDHworks

Department of Work and Pensions: www.dwp.gov.uk

Disabled People Financial Support:
    www.direct.gov.uk/en/DisabledPeople/FinancialSupport/index.htm

Denmark

Overview

Denmark is a constitutional monarchy with a representative democracy. The Danish constitution of 1953 covers the Danish mainland, the Faroe Islands, and Greenland. There are three levels of government: national, regional, and local. Following a reform enacted in January 2007, Denmark now has five regions with elected representations and 98 municipalities/local authorities. The responsibilities of the regions and municipalities are primarily in the areas of social care, education, roads, cultural activities, and health care. In these areas the national government sets frameworks and provides guidelines.

The OHS System

The Ministry of Employment has ultimate authority in matters concerning the working environment, with rules and regulations related to health and safety at work. The key piece of legislation is the Working Environment Act. The Ministry is supported by the Working Environment Authority, an enforcement body that inspects worksites and has the power to punish firms that do not comply with legislation. Punishment includes fines and stop-work orders. Firms can appeal decisions by the Working Environment Authority to a working environment appeal board that consists of representatives from the various social partners. The Ministry of Employment is also supported by the

National Research Centre for the Working Environment, a government research institute that undertakes research on health and safety topics.

The current Working Environment Act was passed in 1999. Its objective is to prevent occupational injury and diseases, and to protect youth and young adults in the labour market. The most recent amendment to the Act was in 2004 in response to the working environment reform adopted by the Danish parliament. This reform includes the introduction of a programme to profile the work environment within firms, an obligation on the part of government to inspect all worksites within a seven-year period, and a duty for firms to seek consulting advice.

The legislation covers how work is performed, workplace design, technical equipment, substances and materials, rest periods, and issues related to workers under the age of 18. The Working Environment Act emphasizes the role of workplace design in protecting workers from having to leave the labour market due to declines in physical and mental health. The Act also emphasizes the role of social and technological progress in changing working conditions, and requires consideration of how best to minimize risks associated with such changes.

The Act is based on the principle of co-operation between employers and workers. The employer is responsible for ensuring a healthy and safe working environment. Workers are obliged to participate in health and safety training, and use protective equipment provided by the employer. All firms with ten or more workers are required to incorporate OHS into their organizational structure, with representation from workers and managers.

Social partnerships play a key role in the Danish OHS system, from appointment to the working environment appeal board to involvement in policy design. Social partners can also participate in the Working Environment Council, which publishes newsletters and guidelines for workplace parties and the general public.

Disability compensation programmes

All employers must purchase workers' compensation insurance covering accidents and short-term effects of exposure to hazardous substances. The insurance does not cover accidents occurring while driving to and from work. All employers must also contribute to the Labour Market Occupational Diseases Fund to cover occupational disease and back injury. The insurance also provides coverage for health care and rehabilitation expenses, wage loss benefits, compensation for permanent impairment, and compensation to families in cases of fatality. Occupational injury and disease claims are reviewed by the National Board of Industrial Injuries, which makes decisions on the compensability of claims and the amount of compensation received.

A modest means-tested disability pension is also provided to adults between the ages of 18 and 64. To qualify, workers must have at least three years of residency in Denmark and their work capacity must be reduced by at least 50%. There are supplements for partial compensation of special expenditures related to physical or mental impairment. If a disability is caused by an occupational injury or disease, workers and their dependants are entitled to compensation.

Health care financing and delivery

Health care financing and delivery are largely public sector responsibilities. For the most part, services are free at the point of delivery, with 85% of health care expenses paid for by taxes. Health care is delivered through the public sector and those providing services are civil servants. Services are coordinated by national government departments and local authorities.

As with the overall structure of government, the health sector has three political and administrative levels—national, regional, and local/municipal. The national level initiates and coordinates programmes and performs an advisory role. The Ministry for the Interior and Health is responsible for all legislation related to health services, and provides guidelines for the provision of health services. Municipalities are responsible for district nursing, public health, school health services, and child dental care. The regions are responsible for hospital services, including specialist care. Each region has the authority to organize health services for their citizens according to regional priorities. All governmental levels are involved in preventive health measures including initiatives in the workplace. The Centre for Public Health, established in 2001, facilitates co-operation between all three levels of government, and serves as a focal point for the development and implementation of new methods for disease prevention and health promotion.

Selected websites on the Danish OHS system

Danish Working Environment Authority: www.at.dk/sw7737.asp
Working Environment Act: www.at.dk/sw12173.asp
National Board of Industrial Injuries: www.ask.dk/sw505.asp
Ministry of Science, Technology and Innovation: www.workindenmark.dk/Industrial_injury
National Research Centre for the Working Environment:
    www.arbejdsmiljoforskning.dk/?lang=en
Ministry of the Interior and Health: www.im.dk/publikationer/health care_in_dk/all.htm

Germany

The OHS system

OHS has a long tradition in Germany beginning in the late nineteenth century. At that time OHS was primarily focused on the avoidance of accidents and the protection of specific worker groups, such as women and children. Today the

German OHS system has a much broader scope, covering the prevention of occupational injury, disease, and OHS health risks. The objectives of the system are to protect workers, improve safety and health, improve working conditions, promote health, improve motivation and job satisfaction, support quality management, and support economic success and competitiveness. Firms also implement their own in-house OHS designed to contribute to health and safety performance while maintaining competitiveness.

Germany is a federation consisting of 16 independent states. The principle of federalism also applies to the OHS system. Nearly all laws in the field of OHS are national laws, decreed by the German Bundestag (the lower house of parliament), usually after a bill has been prepared by the Federal Ministry of Labour and Social Affairs. In some cases, the approval of the Bundesrat (the upper house of parliament) is also necessary in order to pass a bill. Early in the process of preparing a bill, important stakeholders from the various states are consulted. These include the federal states, the umbrella organization (Unfallversicherungsträger) for trade unions, the umbrella organization of the employers, the umbrella associations of the accident insurance institutions, and the professional associations concerned (Fachverbände). In preparing statutory provisions for OHS the German Federal Ministry of Labour and Social Affairs is supported by the Federal Institute for Occupational Safety and Health (Bundesanstalt für Arbeitsschutz und Arbeitsmedizin/BAuA).

The most important OHS statutory provisions are the Occupational Health and Safety Act (Arbeitsschutzgesetz), the Occupational Safety Act (Arbeitssicherheitsgesetz), regulations related to statutory accident insurance within the Seventh Volume of the Code of Social Law (siebtes Sozialgesetzbuch), and Ordinance on Dangerous Substances (Gefahrstoffverordnung).

Though legislation is primarily developed at the national level, it takes into consideration the interests of state-level stakeholders. Stakeholders are responsible for ensuring that national laws and provisions are upheld, hence each state has its own OHS inspectorate (Gewerbeaufsichtsamt or Staatliches Amt für Arbeitsschutz). State inspectorates are responsible for undertaking inspections to ensure that employers are compliant with the law, providing consultative services to employers regarding health and safety issues, and in some cases, initiating necessary interventions.

Employers are responsible for OHS system in their organization. They have a duty to implement necessary measures, taking into account the particular circumstances that might affect their workers. They are also required to appoint safety specialists and company physicians to provide support and advice.

An important principle of the German OHS system is dualism, which refers to two pillars of the system—the state-run system as described above, and the statutory accident insurance and prevention system (workers' compensation), which consists of Berufsgenossenschaften-BG, the provider for industry, Berufsgenossenschaften the provider for agriculture, and accident insurance provided for the public sector. All firms and public sector organizations must be members of one of these insurance programmes. Hence, all workers in Germany are covered by insurance.

Finance and delivery of compensation

Workers' compensation insurance is paid for by employers and coverage extends to all workers. Benefits and services provided by the workers' compensation association include wage replacement benefits, health care services, occupational/vocational services, disability pensions, and nursing care. For health care services, the workers' compensation association negotiates with clinicians and hospitals. Injured and ill workers are often treated in special rehabilitation centres run by the association. During medical treatment and rehabilitation workers receive wage replacement benefits. The first six weeks of benefits are paid for directly by the employer, but after six weeks they are provided by the association. The association is also responsible for social and vocational rehabilitation. In cases of permanent impairment and disability, the association provides continued care as necessary and a disability pension.

Selected websites on the German OHS system

Occupational Health and Safety Information Sources for Germany:
    www.balticseaosh.net/germany/information.shtml
Federal Institute of Occupational Safety and Health:
    www.baua.de/nn_5568/en/Homepage.html__nnn=true
Occupational Safety and Health Accident Insurance: www.hvbg.de/e/pages
BG-Institute for Occupational Safety and Health: http://www.hvbg.de/e/bia
BG-Institute for Occupational Medicine: www.bgfa.ruhr-uni-bochum.de/e/index.php

Australia

Overview

Australia is a federal jurisdiction comprising six states and two territories. However, the precise areas of responsibility between the different levels of government in Australia are becoming increasingly unclear. There is a formal designation of the fields of national government legislative authority in the Commonwealth of Australia Constitution Act. These include the matters of external affairs, customs and excise, trade and commerce, defence, quarantine, immigration, and divorce. Areas of activity outside these designated areas were meant to be the responsibility of the states and territories, including health, policing, education, transport, housing, and environmental regulation. However, as the result of a series of decisions of the High Court of Australia, most restrictions or limits on the powers of the national government have been removed. The national government has, in addition, control over the major areas of tax revenue and, as a result, receives approximately 80% of total tax revenue in Australia. Consequently, many of the major areas formerly under state and territory control, such as health, education and transport, have over time become shared areas of activity.

Arrangements for OHS and workers' compensation in Australia reflect the general pattern of shared federal-state/territorial responsibility. Thus, there are ten schemes, one for each of the six states and two territories, and two national schemes. This is the case for both OHS and workers' compensation. There are specialist OHS statutes covering the mining industry in some states and a specialist workers' compensation scheme for the coal mining industry in New South Wales. With the adoption of 'Robens style' (described later) OHS arrangements in the Australian jurisdictions, there is a considerable degree of homogeneity of the OHS schemes, although jurisdictions still differ significantly in some areas. The ten Australian workers' compensation schemes are, however, characterized by substantial differences, both in terms of their structural features and in relation to benefit entitlements.

In 1985 the National Occupational Health and Safety Commission was established to lead and coordinate national efforts to prevent workplace deaths, injury and disease. It was abolished in 2005 and replaced by the Australian Safety and Compensation Council (ASCC), though this new body was established administratively, rather than under legislation. The responsibility of the ASCC was extended to include workers' compensation as well as OHS. The ASCC, like its predecessor, is a tripartite body, with members currently representing federal, state and territory governments, the Australian Chamber of Commerce and Industry, and the Australian Council of Trade Unions.

OHS legislation

Australian OHS legislation has historically been strongly influenced by the ruling British model. Thus, in the nineteenth century various Australian colonies (later states) essentially copied the British Factories Act legislation (particularly the British Acts of 1878 and 1901). In 1972, the British Robens Report reviewed the weaknesses of the traditional model and proposed alternative legislation. Following this, Australian jurisdictions enacted 'Robens style' legislation, beginning with South Australia in 1972, and today all the state, territory, and national OHS statutes rest upon the Robens model, although some go beyond it. In addition, the challenges of a changing labour market have led jurisdictions to update aspects of their OHS legislation.

Australian OHS statutes adopted the Robens approach of a cascading framework of broad, over-arching general duties, underpinned by more specific and detailed provisions in regulations and codes of practice. The general duties provisions cover the obligations of employers, the self-employed, occupants, manufacturers, suppliers, designers of plants and substances, employees, and some other duty holders. These obligate the duty holder to provide and maintain, as far as is reasonably practicable, a working environment that is safe and without risks to health.

Until the 1990s Australian jurisdictions typically had a host of separate regulations, each relating to a specific hazard. Since the mid-1990s, there has been a move to consolidate regulations. This process has been accompanied by a shift from detailed specification standards within regulations to performance standards, and process and documentation requirements. Currently, the general requirement obligates the duty holder to identify hazards, and assess and control identified risks. Increasingly, duty holders must document their compliance efforts in relation to these responsibilities. Thus, under the Queensland regulatory regime, principal contractors, demolishers, contractors, and subcontractors are required to prepare workplace health and safety work plans before commencing certain types of construction work. Sitting below regulations, but still having the force of law, are codes of practice providing more detailed guidance on hazard identification, and risk assessment processes and procedures.

A significant part of the work of the former National Occupational Health and Safety Commission was to foster and facilitate greater national uniformity, particularly under the aegis of the tripartite National Uniformity Taskforce, established in 1991. It identified key areas for national standards including plant design, occupational noise, manual handling, and major hazardous facilities. The task of achieving greater national uniformity is an expressed priority area for the ASCC.

Enforcement of OHS statutory obligations is the responsibility of an OHS inspectorate. Traditionally, the inspectorate was part of the Department of Labour (or its equivalent). However, there has been a trend in many Australian jurisdictions (including Victoria, New South Wales, and Tasmania) to move the inspectorate into the same regulatory body that has responsibility for the oversight of the worker compensation system. Similarly, there has been a trend towards a more multi-skilled, generalist OHS inspectorate, although differentiated inspectorates are still common in certain areas, such as dangerous goods and construction. OHS inspectors have the ability to issue improvement and prohibition notices, and to initiate prosecutions. In some jurisdictions, inspectors can levy an administrative penalty in the form of an infringement notice.

All Australian OHS legislation provides for some form of worker involvement in OHS matters, particularly as health and safety representatives, and through safety committees. The provisions relating to worker involvement vary considerably. In some jurisdictions, health and safety representatives have quite broad powers, including the rights of inspection, the authority to issue provisional improvement notices, and the authority to issue stop-work orders.

Workers' compensation

There is considerable variation in the nature of Australian workers' compensation arrangements. While all ten schemes provide a system of no-fault statutory benefits underpinned by insurance of workers by premiums or levies compulsorily paid by their employers, this is the only real common feature. The original structure of Australian workers' compensation followed that of the United Kingdom, and was essentially a copy of the English statutes of 1897 and 1906. The system provided relatively limited statutory benefits, access to common law (although in practice this was rarely used) and private insurance underwriting. In terms of underwriting structures, until the mid-1980s the only departure from private underwriting was in Queensland, which in 1916 created a monopoly state fund.

Major changes in workers' compensation structural arrangements occurred in the mid-1980s, largely in response to dramatic increases in insurance premium rates and trade unions' concerns about extended delays in dispute resolution. This led to three jurisdictions (Victoria in 1985, South Australia in 1986, and New South Wales in 1987) to move from private underwriting to monopoly state insurance. Private underwriting of workers' compensation insurance continues to exist in Western Australia, Tasmania, the Northern Territory, the Australian Capital Territory, and the national Seacare scheme, which covers interstate and international merchant shipping.

The changes that occurred in various states in the mid-1980s involved significant restructuring of the form of workers' compensation benefits. In particular, the duration of weekly benefits, which formerly was highly restricted, was extended in some jurisdictions to the standard age of retirement. Similar extensions were also applied to medical and related costs associated with occupational injury.

Other sources of disability compensation

Both workers' compensation and motor vehicle accident compensation are areas of state and territorial responsibility. There are two federal workers' compensation schemes. The first is the Safety, Rehabilitation and Compensation Act 1988 (Comcare), which deals with federal public-sector employment. The second covers seafarers engaged in interstate and overseas trade and commerce under the Seafarers Rehabilitation and Compensation Act 1992. There is no federal motor vehicle accident compensation scheme.

Income security and attendant health care costs in relation to almost all areas of disability, other than that covered by workers' compensation, are the responsibility of the federal government. Income replacement is covered through social security arrangements, primarily the Disability Support Pension (for long-term disability) and Sickness Allowance (for short-term disability). There are other compensation systems, such as the Newstart Allowance (Provisional), the Newstart Allowance (Incapacitated), the Youth Allowance (Incapacitated), and the Mobility Allowance.

Occupational sick leave, paid for by the employer, sits somewhere between the purely federal, and purely state and territory arrangements. It deals with the short-term income loss resulting from injury or disease, but is often governed by a complex interplay of state/territory and federal industrial relations provisions. In terms of private arrangements, it is not uncommon for high-income earners to seek to protect labour-market earnings from the effects of injury, disease, and disability through some form of private disability insurance. Occupational superannuation, formerly a measure largely restricted to limited areas of professional and white collar employment, has become a universal programme as a result of the federal government's concern about the financial impact of having to meet the retirement income needs of an aging population through the federal age pension. While occupational superannuation is primarily a measure dealing with retirement income, many superannuation arrangements, particularly in the public sector, have a disability income component that provides income support if serious injury or disease occurs prior to retirement.

Health care financing and delivery

Australia has a comprehensive national health insurance scheme called Medicare, paid for through a 1.5% levy on taxable income. Individuals are also entitled to purchase private health insurance through competing private carriers. Private health insurance partially reimburses health care and ancillary costs that are not covered by Medicare (for instance, for podiatry or the cost of eye glasses). Private insurance may provide other benefits, such as the ability to gain early access to elective hospital-based procedures for non-life-threatening conditions.

In an attempt to encourage higher income earners to purchase private hospital coverage and, where possible, to use the private system, so reducing the demand on the public system, single people with a taxable annual income in excess of $50,000, and couples and families with a taxable annual income in excess of $100,000 who do not purchase private health care insurance are liable to pay an additional 1% surcharge on their taxable income.

Selected websites on the Australian OHS system

Australian Safety and Compensation Council: www.ascc.gov.au

Occupational Health & Safety Information for Australia:
www.australia.gov.au/Occupational_Health_&_Safety

Disability Support Payments and Allowances:
www.australia.gov.au/Disability_Payments_&_Allowances

Medicare Australia: www.medicareaustralia.gov.au

Chapter 7

Workplace-researcher relationship: early research strategy and avoiding the 'data dearth'

Benjamin C. Amick III, Phil Bigelow, and Donald C. Cole

Introduction

Designing and implementing sound evaluations of occupational health and safety (OHS) interventions is a challenge. Employers are generally uninterested in allowing workers to take time off work to participate in evaluations and many wince at randomization, where some workers receive an intervention and others do not. If it is the intent of researchers also to collect cost, productivity and other data, the challenges become even more daunting: not only must they convince workplace parties (management and labour) to participate, but they must also identify interested employers who have adequate data on health, productivity outcomes, and costs, or who are able and willing to collect it.

Although management might see researchers' need for such data as an added burden, collecting it and conducting reasonable economic evaluations can actually make evaluation studies more interesting to employers. Once the business community sees a good opportunity to develop return-on-investment models with the help of OHS researchers, a new dialogue can emerge between the research community and business, centred on making evidence-based business decisions using scientifically credible evidence.

Likewise, it is false to suppose that unions are opposed to collecting productivity data as part of an OHS study. In truth, labour also has an interest in knowing the resource implications of OHS interventions since this knowledge is useful for contract negotiations, the public and shareholder perceptions of management effectiveness, and the ability of workers to have healthy and successful careers. If researchers fail to consider both the health outcomes and the productivity implications of interventions, stakeholders will not know which interventions have both types of consequence.

Given the diversity of management and labour leadership, we believe there are opportunities to undertake economic evaluations serving the needs of both. In this chapter, we first discuss strategies for successful engagement of stakeholders in OHS interventions and then discuss the special case of small firms. Subsequently, we review options for integrating economics into evaluative studies. The review includes the types of information that might be collected and the study designs that fit different needs. Finally, we present insights gained from a large-scale field intervention on elements we believe will enhance the probability of successfully completing economic evaluations of OHS interventions.

Relationships among stakeholders and researchers

In a recent review of OHS intervention research, Kristensen (2005) emphasized that the primary purpose of workplaces is the production of goods and services, not participation in research. When workplaces do get involved in research, the process typically begins with the company's acceptance of the study, followed by giving the researcher access to the workplace, employees, and documentation. Eventually, the process may lead to the company's wholehearted commitment to the intervention and the study (Kristensen 2005). Kristensen argued that workplaces must benefit from participating in the intervention study if they are to give their full commitment. Researchers therefore stand to gain from investing in intervention methods that combine improved work environment with increased productivity.

Types of stakeholders

Successful economic evaluations of OHS interventions generally require the co-operation of all workplace parties, as well as other interested stakeholders. The primary stakeholders are workers, employers, and unions, while other relevant stakeholders include the families of workers, OHS professionals, business associations, health and safety organizations, health care providers, workers' compensation providers, government agencies, and researchers. At a minimum, good communication with stakeholders is required. If one takes a participatory approach, the challenge increases, since it involves understanding the various perspectives of stakeholders and balancing their needs while maintaining objectivity (Kramer *et al.* 2005).

The degree of interest shown by stakeholders in an intervention and their subsequent participation in it, depend largely on its importance to them. LaMontagne and Needleman (1996) note that an intervention's perceived relevance is a major issue in gaining access and winning co-operation from a study population. Stakeholder involvement is likely to be enhanced further if the research is supported by a respected sponsor and the researchers have established credibility (LaMontagne and Needleman 1996). Considerable background work is often required on the part of researchers to understand social and organizational contexts and to develop relationships before an actual OHS intervention can effectively take place.

Management commitment

Newly introduced programmes are especially dependent on management support as employers bear much of the programme cost, and managers must develop new policies and practices to integrate these programmes into existing business plans. In practical terms, both programme managers (usually OHS professionals) and evaluators/researchers need to keep senior management engaged and committed to the intervention and the evaluation. In an economic evaluation of a mechanical ceiling lifts implementation in a hospital, Yassi and colleagues (1995a,b) emphasized that management commitment and worker participation were critical predictors of (research) success. Other investigators have also emphasized the importance of buy-in by senior management and support from workers (Neumann *et al.* 2002; Gilkey *et al.* 2003a,b; LaMontagne *et al.* 2004; Koningsveld *et al.* 2005).

Gaining and maintaining top management commitment is enhanced when a programme's outcomes fit with the company's values and culture. In a survey of British directors' perspectives on OHS, Smallman and John (2001) reported that sophisticated firms saw OHS not as a separate function, but as part of a broader set of initiatives that target productivity, competitiveness, and profitability. Less progressive companies are also moving away from the idea that OHS is merely the avoidance of adverse health occurrences, towards it being seen as a positive input in their businesses. Economic evaluations can provide support for investing in OHS programmes (Goetzel *et al.* 2005) with the extent of investment dependent on considerations, such as the expected expenditures and potential health benefits (Koningsveld 2005).

There can be discordance between the level of evidence that workplaces require for decision making and that which scientists view as necessary for evidence-based practice. Cole and colleagues (2003) noted that such discordances in cultures of evidence can present barriers to intervention research on musculoskeletal disorders. Management in workplaces must make decisions quickly and sometimes use information that scientists may not even consider (Smallman and John 2001). Once management has embraced an intervention it may be difficult to sustain its interest in its continued evaluation.

Fostering participation

Participatory approaches to organizational change have been advocated for some time (Mann and Neff 1961; Lawler 1975). In 1994, approximately 70% of Fortune 1000 companies in the US used some form of employee participation in OHS programmes (Dumaine 1994). Similarly, stakeholder participation in the evaluation of OHS interventions has been recommended as an effective way to develop generalizable knowledge having benefits for the targeted community (Macaulay *et al.* 1998). Exponential growth in the number of companies implementing participatory ergonomics programmes has occurred in the last decade. Since workers are the most knowledgeable about their own jobs, interventions that effectively utilize their knowledge and insight through participation also increase their sense of ownership of the programme.

The nature of the intervention and the workplace context are important in determining the degree and type of participation. For example, interventions in the design aspects of a process may require employee participation only in the early stages, whereas those that require changing work tasks require worker engagement over a longer term. Degrees of participation can vary at different levels of an organization. Once again, participatory ergonomics provides a good example, since such interventions may involve external agencies within the sector, unions, senior management, supervisors, and workers (Cole *et al.* 2003). The complex relationships, dynamics, and interactions of these players are all part of the intervention and, borrowing from complexity theory, it may be said that the whole is more than the sum of its parts (or in evaluation terms, a programme in its entirety is more effective than the sum of its components).

Providing feedback

A particular challenge in sustaining stakeholder buy-in is the substantial lag time that may exist between a programme's implementation and the realization of its benefits. Maintaining commitment in such cases can be aided by ensuring that management is aware of progress. This can be achieved by presenting intermediate outcomes that are leading indicators for the desired programme effects. An example is to use a measurement tool called the Healthy Workplace Balanced Scorecard, which was developed by researchers to track data on a number of health and safety performance indicators (Robson *et al.* 2005). This Scorecard is based on the popular Balanced Scorecard tool developed to gauge business performance (Kaplan and Norton 1992) and has been developed both by stakeholders and researchers (Robson *et al.* 2005).

The Scorecard consists of four categories of performance indicators (Robson *et al.* 2005): 1) healthy workplace drivers (e.g., OHS leadership, culture, policies and practices); 2) workplace conditions (i.e., physical and psychosocial environments); 3) health outcomes (e.g., absenteeism, injury, pain); and 4) organizational benefits (e.g., employee retention, employee satisfaction, labour efficiency and productivity. In practical applications, the Scorecard can be used as a tool for workplace parties in selecting appropriate indicators for monitoring OHS performance and an intervention's impact on health and productivity. Its use has the potential to facilitate effective communication between all workplace parties, especially if all the stakeholders have participated in the selection of the specific indicators.

Interventions in small establishments

Despite the many challenges of intervention research in small firms, it is worth the effort, since small firms are a disproportionately large number of firms in most industries. Moreover, workers in small firms are at increased risk of occupational injury compared to those in medium and large firms (Gardner *et al.* 1999). Despite this, intervention research in small firms has been sparse, since small firms often have inherent barriers to the implementation of OHS interventions. They include isolation, a lack of OHS knowledge, the high initial cost of interventions (in relation to the firm's budget), conflicting demands on employees, the emphasis on production, and the low frequency of accidents along with the lack of the perception of a need for OHS programmes (Eakin 1992; Holmes *et al.* 1997; Champoux and Brun 2003).

Lack of awareness of the consequences of occupational injury and disease, and the potential gains from their reduction, can sometimes explain the unwillingness of small firms to participate in intervention research. There also may be a mismatch between their perceptions of health risks and the actual risks. Goldenhar *et al.* (1999) used their findings from focus groups of employees and owners in the dry-cleaning industry to suggest that interventions be adapted to influence the perceptions, attitudes, and behaviours of the target population. Research on small companies in Canada has also found that lack of knowledge and recognition of hazards was a major barrier to improving OHS standards and performance in small firms (Champoux and Brun 2003).

Economic evaluations in small firms are often plagued by poor quality data. In small firms, OHS activities that are directly linked to production are more likely to be completed (inspection and maintenance functions), whereas more administrative OHS functions (formal training, written policies and procedures) are not (Champoux and Brun 2003). Data on injury frequency and associated costs are sometimes less reliable in small firms due to a greater tendency to under-report (Champoux and Brun 2003; Kidd *et al.* 2004). Furthermore, insufficient internal resources limit the ability to monitor productivity. These data integrity issues suggest that researchers should be cautious before combining data from small and large firms.

Novel approaches are needed in evaluation research in small firms. There may be an advantage in using existing networks of firms to address the issue of small sample size. In an intervention study of predominantly small residential construction firms in Colorado, partnering with the industry association was found to be effective in overcoming this problem (Gilkey *et al.* 1998). Working with business and industry associations can also be helpful in encouraging sufficient numbers of firms to collect and provide appropriate and reliable data for evaluation purposes. In the aforementioned intervention study in the construction industry, the Homebuilders Association of Metropolitan Denver provided training and assistance in the completion of injury and illness reports (a legislative requirement in the US) and the collection of information on OHS programme expenditures (Gilkey *et al.* 1998, 2003). Other partnership approaches that encourage participation of multiple stakeholders and multiple firms have also proven successful (Materna *et al.* 2002).

Methodological issues in OHS economic evaluation

The overall quality of published intervention studies is not high. Goldenhar and Schulte (1994, 1996) reviewed published OHS interventions and identified several methodological problems that are still to be found in the current OHS literature. The problems included lack of a theoretical framework of analysis, inadequate characterization of the intervention, study designs without comparison groups, selection bias, various problems with measurement, and analytical weaknesses.

They also noted that resource implications were largely ignored in intervention studies (Goldenhar and Schulte 1996).

Disciplines and models

A multi-disciplinary team with expertise in a variety of areas including health and safety, work organization, psychology, engineering, economics, and programme evaluation is often necessary for a successful intervention study. Gaining an understanding of the complexity of the intervention, and its impacts on multiple outcomes and stakeholders is a challenge. A mix of both quantitative and qualitative methods is often required to determine not only whether, but why a programme is successful. Answering 'why' and 'how' questions is perhaps equally as important as answering the question of 'whether' a programme is successful and cost-effective; the lessons learned by addressing the former questions are the basis of future innovation in OHS.

A general model that depicts the various pathways by which OHS interventions can improve health is usually worth developing or adopting as a foundation piece. Figure 7.1 shows one such model in which an individual's health and work demands are the inputs that contribute to individual work role functioning and ultimately to business productivity. Health care can have an effect on health, work role functioning, and business productivity. Work role functioning contributes to organizational performance, which also has an impact on business productivity. Such models help to clarify concepts and can be useful tools in communicating with stakeholders.

Design options

Randomized controlled trials may be the gold standard for intervention studies in general, but recruitment of workplaces even to an intervention group can be exceedingly difficult. Randomization to intervention and control groups is rarely an option in OHS interventions, although there are notable

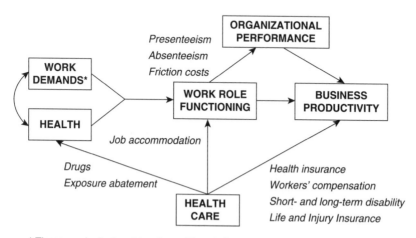

* These can be both paid and unpaid work demands, especially when considering stress-related diseases.

Fig. 7.1 A general model of organizational performance.

exceptions. LaMontagne *et al.* (2004) employed a blind blocked randomization design in which firms were allocated to an intervention involving a health promotion programme alone or to a group receiving the health promotion programme, and an OHS intervention that involved the development of an OHS management system. More commonly, quasi-experimental designs are used (see Chapter 8 for a detailed discussion). Adapting a design to a stakeholder's level of resources and timelines for decision making presents additional challenges.

Sources of productivity data

There are several types and sources of productivity data that might be used in an economic evaluation. Other chapters provide detail on the identification and measurement of costs and consequences (see Chapters 10 and 11). Here, we consider different kinds of measures and data issues associated with various levels within an organization (i.e., the organization as a whole, plant/worksite, department, workgroup, and individual).

At the organizational level, the most common type of information reflecting impacts on health in gross terms relates to absence, often used as a measure of lost productivity. Since these data are generally linked to payroll, they are often readily available from human resource departments. Administrative data on absences are preferred to self-reported absence data, since the latter have questionable validity and reliability (Johns 1994).

At the departmental and workgroup levels, various indicators are routinely used to monitor both productivity (e.g., number of pieces produced per hour) and quality (e.g., percentage of output produced right the first time). In medium-sized manufacturing plants, we have found that production managers are usually willing to share such information, although they may not always appreciate how it may be linked to health. Yet, if research demonstrates that an OHS intervention has an effect on productivity based on a metric already used by an organization, this invariably increases the meaningfulness of the evaluation to that organization. For interventions that have an impact on groups of employees (e.g., slowing down a conveyor belt to facilitate the direction of parcels so that fewer fall off, and thus to reduce the frequency of forward bending and consequential back pain), group measures of productivity are more appropriate than individual measures. In unionized environments, where resistance to individual monitoring may exist, group measures may be the only relevant routinely collected measures.

At the individual level, the gold standard is productivity data obtained through an active monitoring system collecting performance information. Typically, these metrics are used in performance evaluation. For example, in a customer service area call handling time may be a performance indicator, even though it is not necessarily expressed in monetary terms.

Many companies have multiple performance assessment systems. However, the information collected in them may not be valid or reliable. For all in-house administrative data, it is advisable to explore the measures in detail with front-line supervisors. They are generally able to indicate which measures are most valid, reliable and most often used in organizational decision making.

When workplace performance data are unavailable, researchers have relied on self-reported measures. Box 7.1 provides a list of items in self-reported performance measures that are commonly used in human factors and ergonomics research. Although the relationship between business productivity and this suite of measures is not well established, they may be the only option where productivity monitoring data are absent.

Some studies have found that lost productivity that is related to pain occurs mainly when a person is working, rather than through actual absences (Stewart *et al.* 2003). In a clinical trial of the migraine drug sumatriptan, Adelman *et al.* (1996) reported a significant productivity effect only when measuring the lost productivity of a person while at work. Focusing exclusively on productivity losses due to absences may thus result in underestimating the true magnitude of total health-related productivity losses.

At the individual level, 'presenteeism' is increasingly being used to gauge productivity. 'Presenteeism' refers to the level of engagement of an individual while at work. There is a large and heterogeneous literature on presenteeism

Box 7.1 Items commonly used in self-reported productivity measures

Amount of work accomplished

Quality of work accomplished

Meeting deadlines

Frequency of errors

Taking responsibility

Creativity

Getting along with others

Dependability

Overall performance

measures (see e.g., Amick and Gimeno 2007). If these measures are to be useful in economic evaluations, they need to be empirically linked to organizational measures of performance, such as productivity, quality, and profitability. Only a few of them have been linked to existing workplace productivity data with ambiguous results (Burton *et al.* 2001; Bunn *et al.* 2003; Lerner *et al.* 2003; Kessler *et al.* 2003, 2004; Shikiar *et al.* 2004). Nonetheless, presenteeism measures can prove to be important for capturing total productivity.

Ergonomics intervention case study

In this section, we present a case study in which one of us participated and which provides insights into elements that contribute to the success of an evaluation. The study is of a highly adjustable ergonomic chair and an office ergonomics training programme (Amick *et al.* 2003; DeRango *et al.* 2003). The study design was quasi-experimental (i.e., non-randomized controlled), and consisted of three arms: one group receiving a highly adjustable chair and office ergonomics training, a second group receiving training only, and a third control group (this group received training at the end of the study).

The intervention was implemented in a public sector company and was replicated in a private sector company.

Form a transdisciplinary research team

The research team included experts in several disciplines, including economics. Economists with different sub-specialties can be considered for a study depending on the key outcomes of interest. Some possibilities include production economists if productivity improvements due to health are most important, labour economists if lost productivity is emphasized, and health economists if the primary focus is health outcomes.

The team was formed early, and had several retreats to discuss and conceptualize the study design. Developing a comfort level amongst team members takes time, so we ensured sufficient time for team formation in the project timeline. Team members must work together to form a collective sense of the project and a common language. Non-economists must appreciate the data needs of economists and also engage in understanding how the intervention influences productivity. Similarly, economists must appreciate intervention design issues. Thus, all participants are helped to learn new ways of thinking.

Too often economists are asked to participate in an OHS intervention study only after the intervention has been designed and is under way. Consequently, the only input the economist has is in the types of information that can be used in analyses. However, if economists are involved at an earlier stage they can play a pivotal role in the development of a theory of change for the intervention (the pathway through which the intervention ultimately has consequences for the outcomes of interest), as well as assist in identifying companies with sound productivity data.

Ideally, both business and labour representatives should be part of the research team. In the chair study we included a former Director of Health and Safety for a Fortune 500 company as project director. He was the primary link between the research team and the worksite, and was responsible for all briefings. Similarly, in another intervention in a newspaper company, we included a retired trade union activist. Creation of a truly transdisciplinary team will help with representation of the key constituencies.

Build a theory of change

While general theories exist for workplace change, each study should develop an explicit theory of change. Ideally, this should be undertaken earlier rather than later. Working together in formulating the theory contributes to team formation and to the development of a transdisciplinary perspective.

The theory of change used for the chair and ergonomics training intervention is shown in Figure 7.2. We did not expect all productivity improvements to be related to health improvements; rather, productivity was expected to improve in three ways. First, the chair and training would allow workers to be more efficient in their work by organizing their workspace better and improving comfort and satisfaction. Second, productivity might improve because health improved. The effect could be a direct result of health improvements (i.e., more freedom from pain) or indirect through improvements in presenteeism

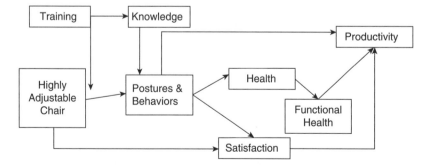

Fig. 7.2 Theory of change for chair and ergonomics training intervention. Source: Amick III BC *et al.*, Effects of an office ergonomic intervention on musculoskeletal symptoms. *Spine* 2003, Lippencott Williams & Wilkins©. Reproduced with permission.

(i.e., engagement). Thirdly, productivity might improve because of reductions in lost work time (i.e., health-related absenteeism).

Identify companies with good productivity data

Over 20 companies were contacted by team members. Contacts were made in multiple ways—through the chair supplier, ergonomists within companies, facility managers within companies, and other business contacts. Each company was approached individually. Bulk letters or emails were not used to solicit interest.

When a company expressed an interest, the management was informed that a requirement for participation was certification by the project economist that their data were sound. As noted, a primary reason for economists to be involved early in a project is for the review of productivity data. Invariably, the primary reason a company was excluded from consideration was due to inadequate productivity data.

An important consideration when evaluating productivity data is the availability of other relevant data, such as work hours. While it is common to assume that an average number of hours are worked per week, a stronger analysis would use data on actual hours worked and actual hours absent.

Gain company trust and commitment

Once a company has expressed interest, and the soundness of its productivity data has been confirmed, the next step is to gain a formal participation agreement. A letter of support from the company will be necessary for approval by a human subjects ethics review committee. It is also advisable to have a signed formal agreement from a senior manager listing the types of data to be provided by the company, constraints on releasing company information in publications, deliverables to the company, and steps to be taken to protect workers. Such a document will formalize top management's interest in participating. If top management's interest cannot be secured, the intervention should not be undertaken, despite any interest other workplace parties might have, so it is important to work with key workplace contacts early on to secure broad-based support from workplace parties (i.e., unions, middle management, and, most importantly, top management).

Having at least one internal champion is critical. The champion is an active advocate for the project. This person can play a key communications role, providing regular updates to management. The champion can also be helpful in relationships with supervisors during project implementation, and with human resources and systems staff when trying to secure personnel and productivity data.

In the chair and ergonomics intervention study several activities were designed to build interest, trust and commitment. We developed a '30-second elevator speech', so that the study could be quickly communicated to workplace parties. We also developed a short visual presentation providing a project overview, the time commitments required, the types of data the business needed to provide, and the deliverables to the company on a specific timeline. We also prepared a one-page project summary. Any of these could be used by team members when speaking with individuals at potential study sites or by internal champions in communications with workplace parties.

It is also important to assure management and unions that everyone at the worksite will have an opportunity to participate in the intervention and that all participants will receive some benefits. In our study, the company received 100 chairs free of charge (valued at $US 600 per chair) and a customized ergonomics training programme for staff that included instructions with site-specific photographs. The project team trained the internal champion to deliver the session. The company also received an ergonomics assessment of the work-stations of all workers participating in the study.

Budgeting sufficient funds for the up-front development work, products, and interactions can, in our experience, substantially increase participation rates at worksites. Many OHS studies have low participation rates, with conse-quential low statistical power, validity and generalizability. In our study, the up-front strategies appeared to be successful. We had very high participation rates (between 70 and 85%) and very little loss to follow-up (less than 5%).

Link productivity data to health data

Linking micro-level health and productivity data can substantially increase the relevance of a study, but requires careful planning, since ethics review committees need strong assurance that the privacy of participants will be pro-tected. In our chair study, data were collected from one year before the interven-tion to one year after. We were able to link health and productivity data and found that use of the chair with the training intervention led to a reduction in musculoskeletal symptoms growth and increased productivity.

Provide timely information back to stakeholders

Employers and researchers usually work on different timelines. An important part of sustaining trust and commitment is the provision of findings and progress updates throughout the project. Management and labour require early results and internal champions can use intermediate results to good effect in their communications with workplace parties. In our study, we conducted workstation assessments pre-intervention and provided feedback to the participants. The training programme was delivered to the control group as a product during the post-intervention phase. The key results, including the return on investment, were provided only a few months after the project's end. An additional benefit of providing timely information to workplace parties is that businesses may communicate their experiences to others, thus opening doors for researchers to new workplaces that could be sites for future intervention evaluations.

Foster sustainability and limit loss to follow-up

A long-term intervention can have the problem of limited participation and substantial loss to follow-up. This is particularly a concern with participants in the control group. The following are some suggestions based on efforts we undertook to address these issues:

- Brief senior management and all involved supervisors about the study.
- Have senior management and senior labour officials send out a letter to all employees announcing the collaboration.
- To assist with implementation, have supervisors hold a series of question-and-answer sessions with workers.
- Set up a series of meetings throughout the project to brief stakeholders. Some of these briefings may be conducted by the internal champion.
- Provide a meaningful reward for participation. What is perceived as a meaningful incentive will vary from worksite to worksite, but the rewards need not be extravagant. Even small tokens of appreciation for participants' time, such as lunch tickets, can be sufficient.

Summary and recommendations

Both the literature and our personal experiences underscore the importance of the front-end developmental work to ensuring the success of an OHS intervention study. Forming a team early in the process and including an economist at the outset of the study planning process are recommended. Also, researchers are encouraged to consider including business and labour representation in the team. The early formation of a team will provide an opportunity to develop a collective sense of the project, which in turn will enhance communication amongst the team members.

Use existing networks of firms and industry associations to help identify appropriate candidate firms and worksites for intervention. Finding a firm with good administrative data and an interest in the project is fundamental. The economist in the team should play a central role in evaluating the appropriateness of available data and productivity data in particular. Though micro-level productivity and performance data are the gold standard, data at various levels of aggregation may be sufficient. Explore data validity and reliability with front-line supervisors who work with the data on a regular basis. In cases where data are not available, the team might consider collecting self-report data. Once a firm is identified, we strongly recommend developing a formal agreement jointly signed by senior management and the principal investigator of the research team. It should detain data sharing arrangements and conditions, publication requirements, deliverables to the company, and worker privacy protection.

In general, the study design should be customized to suit the context. It should not be 'one size fits all'. Factors such as the firm size, types of data available, and culture of the firm all bear on appropriate design. Small organizations present unique challenges. Isolation, limited resources and data, lack of knowledge of OHS issues, conflicting demands on time, and emphasis on production, all present barriers. Part of the customization of the design might include a theory of change specific to the study at hand. Researchers are encouraged to investigate the issue of presenteeism at the firm, as it might be equally as relevant as absenteeism, and at-work performance may be significantly influenced by the intervention.

Building a strong relationship with workplace parties requires ongoing efforts from beginning to end. At the front end, the research team will need to demonstrate the merits of participation to workplace parties. It is, indeed, reasonable to promote evidence-informed decision making both to management and workers, since it can enhance business performance, as well as health and safety. Full commitment from workplace parties may not happen immediately; it requires ongoing relationship building. It helps to identify a champion within the firm who can be a spokesperson for the project. Fostering participation at various levels of the firm can help. Meaningful rewards should be provided to all participants and, ultimately, all workers should have an opportunity to benefit, even those in control groups (e.g., benefits, such as training, can be provided at the end of the study). Ongoing updates and reporting on intermediate outcomes to management and workers are necessary to ensure sustained commitment, since research time lines can be quite different from those of managers and workers.

Part 2

Specific topics

Chapter 8

Study design

William Gnam, Lynda Robson, and Thomas Kohstall

Introduction

This chapter considers issues of study design in determining the effectiveness of occupational health and safety (OHS) interventions. We focus on how study design may affect the validity of an estimate of the net intervention effect (defined as the difference between the outcomes of the intervention and those of the alternative to which it is being compared). This discussion is directly relevant to economic evaluations since estimates of net value are derived from estimates of effects. We cover overall design issues but not other important specific aspects such as recruitment or data collection (see Chapter 7 for details).

Study design considerations cannot be abstracted from the nature of the intervention to be evaluated and the context into which it is introduced. The theoretical basis for selecting an intervention, the method and location of its implementation, the potential health and other consequences that arise from the intervention, and the likely timing of these events should all be considerations when designing a study. These are usually made collaboratively by the research team and, in particular, require input from researchers with expertise in implementing the intervention in the target work population. An OHS economic analyst will typically not be directly responsible for the selection of the design of an intervention evaluation and is more likely to seek accommodation of economic evaluation priorities through indirect methods (Goldenhar *et al.* 2001).

There is considerable overlap between the data needs of an economic evaluation and those of an effectiveness evaluation. However, these needs diverge in several respects. First, an economic evaluation often requires data from several sources synthesized through modelling in order to determine the net effect of interest. Secondly, in an economic evaluation one is usually interested in determining the net effect of the entire stream of consequences of the intervention, including productivity effects. Intervention effectiveness research, on the other hand, may focus on a narrower set of outcomes (e.g., only health outcomes). Thirdly, with randomized designs, an economic evaluation usually focuses on an estimation of the net intervention effect according to randomization assignment (also termed the 'intention to treat' estimate), even if some individuals randomized to the control group receive the intervention and some randomized to the intervention group do not receive the intervention (Mandelblatt *et al.* 1996). Some effectiveness evaluations take this same approach, but others focus on the net effect of the intervention on those study participants who actually receive it. This is termed an efficacy evaluation (see Box 8.1). Finally, an economic evaluation uses data on the final outcomes of an intervention (at one or more specific time intervals following an intervention). An effectiveness evaluation, by contrast, may also involve data on the implementation of the intervention and on its intermediate outcomes.

For the purposes of exposition, we assume that the economic analyst seeks to obtain an estimate of the consequences of an intervention that is well defined and for which there is at least some preliminary evidence to support the feasibility of its implementation in a defined population of workers. We further assume that the analyst can consider the full range of available opportunities for obtaining the estimate, including any of prospective participation in a study involving primary data collection, secondary analysis of existing data sources, and synthesis of other studies. From this stance, the economic analyst, as part of the research team, ought to consider the array of feasible designs and help choose amongst them.

Box 8.1 Some essential definitions

Internal validity: the legitimacy with which we infer that a given intervention did (or did not) produce the observed effects on the outcome variables.

External validity: the legitimacy with which an intervention's observed effects can be generalized from the study subjects to a target population undergoing the intervention under normal circumstances.

Effectiveness: the extent to which an intervention has the desired outcome. Effectiveness sometimes has the more specific meaning of the extent to which an intervention has the desired outcome under normal circumstances, which may be less than ideal.

Efficacy: the extent to which an intervention has the desired outcome under ideal circumstances.

Objectives of study design for economic evaluations

When planning a study design for a particular intervention evaluation, the economic analyst determines how best to obtain an estimate of the net effect that is both internally and externally valid (see Box 8.1), under constraints such as time, expense, data availability, and ethical considerations. Solutions to this problem are not readily evident in the case of OHS interventions, since there is often a trade-off between internal and external validity. Furthermore, it might take several years before all the health and other consequences that are relevant to the economic analysis can be observed.

Internal validity depends on numerous factors, including the comparability of the intervention and comparison group(s), the quality of the measurement of study variables, and the appropriateness of the statistical analysis. Internal validity can often be optimized using a randomized controlled trial (RCT) design. However, the procedures of subject selection and randomization involved in this design can yield samples of workers or workplaces that are unrepresentative of the broader populations to which an economic evaluation typically extends. Similarly, the procedures of stringent intervention implementation and intensive measurement, often involved in RCTs, especially those examining efficacy, are likely to overestimate the effects realizable in normal practice.

An emphasis on internal validity was a marked characteristic of the early practice of evidence-based medicine (Laupacis *et al.* 1992) and hierarchies of evidence were established, which used internal validity as the principal criterion. Later approaches have been both more pragmatic and more pluralistic in their selection of criteria, and the consequential ranking of studies, allowing some to contribute to a better understanding of an intervention's potential and others to forecast how effective it was likely to be in routine practice (Andrews 1993; National Institute for Clinical Excellence 2005).

Study designs

Table 8.1 provides a classification of study designs available for use in OHS intervention evaluations. This list is not exhaustive, and excludes some quasi-experimental designs found in social science research that are uncommon or even non-existent in OHS intervention studies (see Shadish *et al.* 2002). Aided by a recent design classification algorithm (Zaza *et al.* 2000), the classification of studies adapts the ones described in the classic text of Cook and Campbell (1979), so as to include the common epidemiological designs of cohort and case-control. Besides the design categories of experimental and quasi-experimental, Cook and Campbell (1979) also included the non-experimental design category.

Table 8.1 Feasible study designs for determining net intervention effect.

Single study designs	Synthetic study designs
Experimental designs	Meta-analysis
Randomized controlled trial (RCT)	Consensus panel
Cluster RCT	
Quasi-experimental designs	
Non-equivalent control group	
Interrupted time series	
Cohort	
Case-control	
Before–after	

An example in this category is a correlational study between variables in a one-shot survey. Non-experimental designs are not included here because of their inability to yield valid quantitative measures of effectiveness. See Shadish *et al.* (2002) for further explication of non-experimental designs.

Experimental designs

Randomized controlled trial

Statistical theory suggests that the optimal study design for internal validity is one in which individual subjects participating in the study are randomly allocated to one or more intervention groups and a control group (Fisher 1973). Randomization ensures that the characteristics of individuals have been allocated to groups in an unbiased manner. Moreover, as the number of individuals allocated becomes larger, the groups become more likely to be balanced in both observed and unobserved characteristics. Randomization, therefore, enhances the comparability of the intervention and control groups, and provides a more valid basis for inferring that the intervention actually caused the differences in the outcomes observed between groups (Rubin 1991).

Another advantage of RCTs is that the groups being compared are contemporaneous. Such control groups are preferred to the use of historical control groups, since the former are more likely to avoid the bias created by co-interventions or secular changes over time in work environments.

Despite the advantages of high levels of internal validity, reviews of OHS intervention research (Shannon *et al.* 1999; Goldenhar *et al.* 2001) found that intervention research using experimental designs is rare, although they are sometimes used in workplace back-injury prevention programmes, return to work programmes, workplace stress interventions, and occupational hygiene interventions. A review of the nascent literature on the cost-effectiveness of OHS interventions in the health care sector indicated that economic evaluations based on experimental designs are also rare (Niven 2002).

Amongst the disadvantages of designs using randomization are: study subject selection limiting external validity, poor correspondence between an intervention under experimental conditions and the intervention in real occupational settings, and their generally higher costs.

A further disadvantage for economic evaluation includes the limited time horizon of many RCTs, since adverse or costly consequences important to the economic evaluation may be rare, or occur only months or years after the intervention has been implemented.

In OHS settings, experimental study designs face other obstacles that, while not unique to these settings, can easily occur in occupational contexts. Following the classic discussion of Cook and Campbell (1979), these disadvantages can be classified under statistical power, the choice of units for randomization, study group contamination, and compensatory treatment in the control units. In occupational settings, outcomes such as occupational injuries can be relatively rare events from a statistical perspective, requiring either large sample sizes or prolonged follow-up intervals, or both. The scale and duration of effort to collect these data may not be feasible in occupational settings. Choice of the study design in OHS interventions is frequently complicated by the fact that many interventions affect more than one individual, or that spill-over effects occur in which one or more workers will influence the behaviour and outcomes of other workers at the same site who may be members of the control group. Compensatory treatment in the control group may occur if the intervention appears desirable, leading those assigned to control conditions to balk at their assignment, or to seek some kind of co-intervention. Pressure for control groups to receive the study intervention may come from workers, supervisors, company administrators, or company medical officers.

Cluster randomized controlled trial

One way of addressing a concern about spill-over is to randomize at a higher level of aggregation, such as the work group or work site, using a design known as cluster randomization. Cluster randomization reduces statistical power and has its own logistical challenges, but is an option worth entertaining in situations where contamination is likely to occur, as when there is close proximity between subjects receiving the intervention and controls.

Quasi-experimental designs

In quasi-experiments, the assignment of exposure to the intervention being evaluated is achieved by means other than randomization. The first type of quasi-experimental design discussed below resembles a RCT by involving distinct, contemporaneous comparison groups, whereas other quasi-experimental designs do not have this feature.

Non-equivalent control group

In the non-equivalent control group design (also known as a non-randomized trial), study subjects are intentionally assigned for purposes of evaluation to exposure or control conditions through a non-random means by an investigator, administrator, or other decision maker. Although the comparison group generally does not resemble the intervention group in all characteristics, it is desirable that groups be comparable, especially on factors related to the outcomes of the study. In some cases, the investigator may be able to create groups using a process that ensures they are matched on such factors. Whenever possible, the intervention group and non-equivalent control group should be identified before the intervention so that baseline measures can be taken.

This design can have advantages over randomized trials in terms of feasibility, while the non-random assignment of units to the intervention or control condition may allow the study to more closely emulate real workplace conditions. These advantages come, however, at the cost of introducing a potential for bias due to confounding (i.e., when pre-existing differences in the groups instead of the intervention cause the observed effect), particularly if assignment to the intervention or comparison group is related to the outcome (e.g., high-injury units are assigned to the OHS intervention condition). Methods of dealing with this problem (e.g., stratification, multiple regression, propensity scores) and their limitations are discussed in Deeks et al. (2003).

Interrupted time series

The simple interrupted time series design (Cook and Campbell 1979; Cook et al. 1990; Shadish et al. 2002) involves multiple measurements of the outcome in a group before and after the implementation of an intervention. If the change in the outcome variable following the intervention is significant, an effect of the intervention can be inferred, assuming that there is an absence of extraneous influences on the outcome. Recent advances in time series methods allow investigators to test for changes in outcome following an intervention, even when the lag between the intervention and its outcome is unknown. An advantage of this design is that the group being studied typically has real-world relevance (e.g., work group, work site, or jurisdiction).

Furthermore, because the observed group is defined by a setting, tracking of every member of the group, as in cohort studies, is not required; turnover of members is expected (although a large amount of it threatens internal validity). Of major concern with this design is the impact of extraneous influences. The addition of a strategically chosen non-equivalent control group to the design (i.e., time series with non-equivalent control) can consequently strengthen validity considerably.

Cohort

In observational cohort studies, a defined study population that is initially free of the outcome under investigation is followed longitudinally to compare the rates of occurrence of the outcome of interest in subgroups. In the context of intervention studies the subgroups of interest in the cohort are defined by their exposure or lack of it to the intervention of interest. Unlike the non-equivalent group design, exposure to the intervention is not by a decision maker for the purposes of evaluation; rather, it is through natural processes, e.g., self-selection. Longitudinal follow-up may be prospective, such that data collection is planned on the basis of an evaluation research question. Follow-up could also be retrospective, in which case data collection has taken place for another reason and is then later used for evaluative purposes.

Observational cohorts have the potential for stronger external validity than RCTs, since they typically comprise a broader and more representative sample of the population of interest and often involve interventions delivered in real-world settings. However, the economic analyst needs to pay attention to how the subgroups are defined. If defined as the actual exposure to the intervention, as is often the case in cohort studies, then the effect estimate might be one of efficacy, rather than true effectiveness. The major disadvantage of observational cohort studies is possible confounding due to pre-existing differences between intervention and comparison groups in factors affecting the outcome under consideration. In comparison to RCTs or other quasi-experimental designs where the investigator assigns the intervention, observational cohort studies are generally more vulnerable to selection effects as there may be considerable uncertainty about how the intervention was assigned among workers.

Understanding the assignment mechanism of subjects to the intervention and anticipating likely sources of bias is important in devising strategies to reduce it. Bias can sometimes be reduced through the use of statistical modelling procedures, most commonly through covariance adjustment (as in multiple linear or logistic regression modelling), or by stratifying (also known in statistical literature as sub-classifying) the analysis by known potential confounding risk factors (Zwerling et al. 1997). If multiple confounding risk factors for the outcome are present, stratification becomes impractical and covariance adjustment is commonly used. While covariance adjustment through standard statistical modelling may reduce bias, it relies on assumptions about functional form. It can also exacerbate underlying bias in ways that are hard to detect by introducing unwarranted extrapolation, as when the intervention and comparison groups overlap minimally on confounding risk factors (Little and Rubin 2000).

Advances in statistical methods of multivariate matching [such as propensity scores (Rosenbaum and Rubin 1983)] provide new methods of reducing bias when estimating net intervention effects. They include diagnostic procedures to identify non-overlapping observational subgroups on observed confounding factors (Zwerling *et al.* 1997). These matching methods are often used in conjunction with standard covariance adjustment (Dehejia and Wahba 1999). Some methods texts on matching and other observational study methods have recommended replicating the analysis with multiple independent comparison groups (Rosenbaum 1995).

Case-control

In case-control studies, subjects are chosen because they do (the cases) or do not (the controls) exhibit the outcome of interest. Exposure to the intervention is then determined retrospectively. Case-control designs have the advantages of not requiring follow-up and of being able to efficiently sample large numbers of individuals having the outcome of interest. However, like cohort studies, internal validity is subject to bias from confounding factors. Recall bias may also occur if subjects with the outcome are more or less likely to recall having the intervention. Case-control studies are also vulnerable to bias if investigators exert more or less effort to elicit recall of an intervention in controls compared with cases. Using cases and controls from a large cohort study (a nested case-control design) may reduce these problems because data on exposure have already been collected (Rothman and Greenland 1998).

Before–after

In the before–after design, a single occupational group has an outcome measured before and after an intervention, with its change in the outcome's magnitude then taken as the intervention effect. This design is frequently used in safety studies and has also served as the basis for some OHS economic evaluations (Niven 2002).

This design involves several major threats to internal validity, leading Cook and Campbell (1979) to consider it to be a generally (but not invariably) 'uninterpretable' quasi-experimental design. The most pronounced usual threats in OHS studies of this type are co-interventions (initiatives that are directed toward the OHS outcome of interest beside the intervention being examined) and changes in the external environment that are unrelated to the intervention, but which influence the outcome (i.e., history effects). Examples of the latter include changes in policies, management, personnel or technology in a workplace. Other threats include natural changes in the study subjects over time not related to the intervention (maturation), artefacts created by pre-intervention measurement itself (a testing effect), changes in the reporting of outcomes brought about by the intervention, and regression to the mean if extreme individuals or groups are chosen for the study. Many of these threats are reduced when the effects of the intervention can be observed almost immediately, as when exposure to a chemical hazard is immediately reduced by a substitution or engineering intervention. For most OHS interventions, however, especially when health is the outcome of interest, a simple pre–post design is not sufficient to establish internally valid estimates of intervention effects.

Strengthening quasi-experimental designs

The previous discussion indicated a number of ways in which quasi-experimental designs can be strengthened: inclusion of a control group, especially a matched group; collecting data at multiple time points pre- and post-intervention; and statistical control at the analysis stage. Other strategies are elaborated in Shadish *et al.* (2002). They include switching replication (when the intervention is later introduced to a non-equivalent control group), removed treatment (suitable for interventions without lasting effects), repeated treatments (where an intervention is reintroduced after removal), and measuring non-equivalent dependent variables. The latter technique involves measuring two different types of outcomes [e.g., different types of injuries as in Mohr and Clemmer (1989)]—one expected to change because of the intervention, the other not. Finally, the use of independent data to address a particular threat to internal validity might also be used.

Synthesis study designs

Meta-analysis

In meta-analysis, systematic procedures are used to identify, compile, and summarize the results of independent studies of intervention effects. Combining data can increase statistical power to detect intervention effects and enhance the precision of effect size estimates.

Details of meta-analytic procedures are not described here, but are accessible in many publications (e.g., Cooper and Hedges 1994; Egger *et al.* 2003). While there is consensus regarding some aspects of meta-analysis methodology, debate persists, for example, over the role of unpublished data in the meta-analysis, the optimal functional form of the statistical meta-analytical model, and the appropriateness of Bayesian methods. Uncertainty often exists about whether one or more marginal studies should be included.

For the economist, an important question is whether meta-analysis ought to be routinely preferred over single studies when there are several studies reporting on the same outcome. Meta-analysis is generally preferred in situations where there are conflicting studies or when combining information from several studies will improve external validity. The optimal choice is less clear when studies differ significantly in methodological quality or when one study's quality clearly surpasses that of all others.

Consensus panel

Expert opinion is occasionally elicited through a structured means (such as Delphi methods or systematic elicitation of group or individual judgments) to estimate the value of parameters for which other data sources are unavailable. These methods are generally not recommended for providing estimates of the main effects of interventions. They are subject to too many unknown biases, the seriousness of which could be considerable.

Choosing between designs

The prevalence of many considerations when choosing a study design suggests that there is no universal design hierarchy to guide the economist and the research team. In many practical situations the choice of design may be limited by time, resources, the availability of pre-existing data sources, or by trials whose design features are dominated by the requirements of creating valid inferences about intervention efficacy.

Experimental designs should be preferred where high-quality RCTs are possible and other data sources are available if needed to allow the analyst to model adequate time horizons and to generalize. However, the stronger quasi-experimental designs represent an alternative that may be preferred under some circumstances. With an appreciation of the relative strengths and weaknesses of available designs and a thorough survey of the data sources and opportunities available, the research team will be well-placed to choose an appropriate design.

Recommendations

To summarize, the presence of many factors to be considered when choosing a study design implies that there is no universal design hierarchy to guide the economist and the research team. In general, most evaluations require a synthesis of data from two or more sources. Our key recommendations are as follows:

- Choose the study design that best ensures that an estimate of net outcomes is both internally and externally valid.

- Be explicit in the research report about the reasons for the choice of study design.

- Consider an experimental design. This design is generally preferred for its internal validity, particularly if issues of external validity can be adequately addressed through synthesis.

- Consider as an alternative to an experimental design, a quasi-experimental design with features enhancing internal validity, such as matched contemporaneous control groups, data collection at multiple points in time pre- and post-intervention, and statistical adjustments. Designs with these features are strong alternatives to experimental designs and under some circumstances represent the preferred approaches.

- Avoid, if possible, case-control studies and before–after designs. These designs introduce severe threats to internal validity of the estimated intervention effect, and are rarely satisfactory as a primary source of evidence for economic evaluations.

Chapter 9

Kind of analysis and decision rule

Jeffrey S. Hoch and Carolyn S. Dewa

Introduction

To advance and help to standardize the methods of economic evaluation in the occupational health and safety (OHS) field we describe the key principles of economic evaluation. We focus on two key considerations related to the evaluation of OHS interventions: the kind of analysis that should be done and the ways in which the results should be used to make decisions.

Statement of the problem: Justification for economic analysis

Economics is about how best to use scarce resources. Traditional economic models pose an optimization problem and derive decision rules that prescribe how to use scarce resources optimally. An objective function is postulated along with various constraints. The solution to the constrained optimization problem identifies how best to use scarce resources given the perspective embodied in the objective function and the constraints.

Profit maximization as an objective

Consider a profit maximizing firm deciding on how much to invest in an OHS programme that increases the productivity of workers, such as a programme to reduce depression in the workplace. Extra revenue from the programme would come from additional productivity (e.g., through reductions in absenteeism and presenteeism). The costs of the programme include those of detecting and treating depression, employee assistance and counselling. The optimal size of the programme is the level at which the marginal revenue from the programme is equal to its marginal costs. This is often symbolized as $\Delta R = \Delta C$ (see Appendix 1 for a detailed example).

Figure 9.1 elaborates on the $\Delta R = \Delta C$ equation. The diagram depicts the total revenue (TR) and total cost (TC) curves for a hypothetical employer. When the slopes of the revenue and cost curves are equal, $\Delta R = \Delta C$. It is clear that the two curves intersect at two places: 1) when the programme level is between 0 and 1, and 2) when the programme level is between 3 and 4.

These indicate instances where TR = TC. However, $\Delta R = \Delta C$ at only one point. As the programme level goes from 2 to 3, ΔR goes from 10.7 to 10.4, while ΔC goes from 4.7 to 12.7. Thus, somewhere between 2 and 3 (near 2.3 to be more exact), $\Delta R = \Delta C$ and this indicates the optimal level of the OHS programme from a profit maximizing perspective.

Health maximization as an objective

Some organizations may not have profit maximization as their objective, but rather health maximization. For example, a public workers' compensation authority may have the maximization of worker health as their objective. At the same time, a fixed budget may constrain the authority's spending ability.

In the most general sense, the authority could consider m different programmes (say $x_1, ..., x_m$). One programme may be the provision of safety

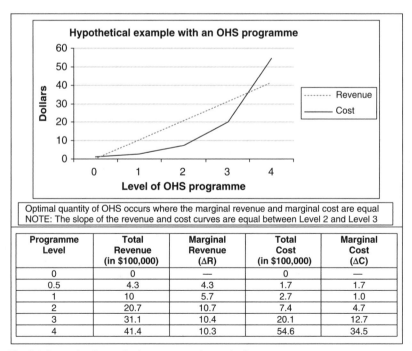

Optimal quantity of OHS occurs where the marginal revenue and marginal cost are equal
NOTE: The slope of the revenue and cost curves are equal between Level 2 and Level 3

Programme Level	Total Revenue (in $100,000)	Marginal Revenue (ΔR)	Total Cost (in $100,000)	Marginal Cost (ΔC)
0	0	—	0	—
0.5	4.3	4.3	1.7	1.7
1	10	5.7	2.7	1.0
2	20.7	10.7	7.4	4.7
3	31.1	10.4	20.1	12.7
4	41.4	10.3	54.6	34.5

Fig. 9.1 Example of marginal revenue and marginal cost curves.

consultations; it can be compared with other uses of the money that also improve the health of workers. This type of problem is called constrained optimization because the fixed budget constrains the ability to provide an OHS programme and all other programmes, which we shall refer to as OTHER.

Figure 9.2 illustrates the solution to a constrained optimization problem using a hypothetical example of the relationship between marginal benefit, marginal cost and the optimal amount of an OHS programme. We use Quality-Adjusted Life-Years (QALYs) as a proxy for health. The optimal point occurs when the slopes of the budget constraint and the QALY curve are equal. This happens when two conditions are met. The first is that the ratio of the extra cost to the extra QALYs (from the OHS programme under consideration) equals the ratio of the extra cost to the extra QALYs (from the OTHER programmes). The second condition (derived in Appendix 2) indicates that the extra cost per extra QALY must be no more than the willingness to pay (λ) for an additional QALY.

The optimal decision rule for the health maximization scenario is similar to that for the for-profit firm. In both cases, OHS should be invested in until the

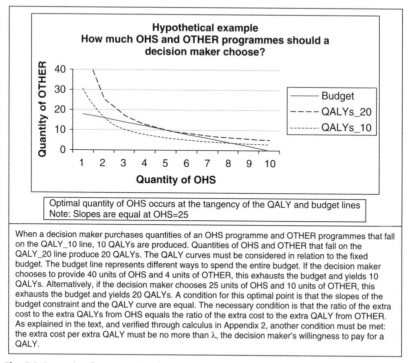

Optimal quantity of OHS occurs at the tangency of the QALY and budget lines
Note: Slopes are equal at OHS=25

When a decision maker purchases quantities of an OHS programme and OTHER programmes that fall on the QALY_10 line, 10 QALYs are produced. Quantities of OHS and OTHER that fall on the QALY_20 line produce 20 QALYs. The QALY curves must be considered in relation to the fixed budget. The budget line represents different ways to spend the entire budget. If the decision maker chooses to provide 40 units of OHS and 4 units of OTHER, this exhausts the budget and yields 10 QALYs. Alternatively, if the decision maker chooses 25 units of OHS and 10 units of OTHER, this exhausts the budget and yields 20 QALYs. A condition for this optimal point is that the slopes of the budget constraint and the QALY curve are equal. The necessary condition is that the ratio of the extra cost to the extra QALYs from OHS equals the ratio of the extra cost to the extra QALY from OTHER. As explained in the text, and verified through calculus in Appendix 2, another condition must be met: the extra cost per extra QALY must be no more than λ, the decision maker's willingness to pay for a QALY.

Fig. 9.2 Example of a constrained optimization problem.

extra benefit (ΔB) equals the extra cost (ΔC), though when outcomes are measured in a non-monetary unit, they are generally described as 'extra effects' (ΔE), rather than 'extra benefits'. The latter term is generally used when consequences are in monetary units. For the for-profit firm, the benefit is measured in revenue (i.e., $\Delta B \equiv \Delta R$); however, in the case of health maximization, the benefit is measured in a non-monetary format (i.e., extra QALYs). To be able to compare the consequences of OHS with ΔC (which is measured in monetary units), extra QALYs must be converted into monetary units as well. The monetary value of the extra QALYs is calculated as the product of λ times the extra QALYs from OHS programme, where λ is the willingness to pay for, or monetary value of an extra QALY. However, the λ used to convert the extra non-monetary outcome into a monetary equivalent is generally unknown in practice and there may be good reasons for leaving it as an open question that is to be determined by decision makers when weighing all the various factors involved in decisions about such investments.

Types of economic evaluation

The solutions to the previous optimization problems are based on theory. In practice it is not always easy to identify the objective, the constraints, or the costs. The answers will certainly depend on who is making the decision, which in turn determines the perspective. What the theory can do is to make clear the kind of factors that must be considered (preferably explicitly) and thereby identify the kinds of information that can inform the decision maker and, one conjectures, that will lead to better decisions.

Decisions always involve trade-offs. To invest more in X, one must invest less in Y. Different ways of describing these trade-offs have given rise to different types of economic evaluation. Each involves costs measured in monetary terms; the key difference between them lies in how health, and other consequences or outcomes are measured (we shall treat 'consequences' and 'outcomes' as synonyms). Choosing the appropriate kind of evaluation to use in OHS can be a challenge because of the multiple stakeholders involved (see Chapter 2). A key consideration is the trade-off that matters most to the decision maker. Table 9.1 presents the different types of economic evaluations with their corresponding sample results, decision rules, advantages and limitations. We elaborate on each type below.

Cost–benefit analysis (CBA)

In cost–benefit analysis (CBA) all outcomes are measured in monetary units. Having both costs and benefits measured in the same units facilitates comparison with alternatives uses of resources that are not in the OHS arena, particularly

Table 9.1 Different types of economic evaluations and their characteristics.

Kind of economic evaluation	Sample result (study example)	Decision rule for selecting the programme	Advantages	Limitations
Cost–benefit analysis (CBA)	Extra benefits are ΔB and extra costs are ΔC. (Englander et al. 1996)	If $\Delta B > \Delta C$	Both benefits and costs are valued in monetary units	May be difficult to obtain objective monetary values for non-monetary consequences
Cost-effectiveness analysis (CEA)	Extra cost per depression free day is $22 (Simon et al. 2001)	If there is money in the budget and if a depression free day is felt to be worth at least $22	Outcomes are measured in natural units to facilitate under-standing of health effects	Different outcomes from different programmes are not easily comparable
Cost–utility analysis (CUA)	Extra cost per QALY is $57,000 (Chodick et al. 2002)	If there is money in the budget and if a QALY is felt to be worth at least $57,000	QALYs make all health programmes comparable	There are many ways to estimate a QALY and different ways can yield different answers.
Cost-minimization analysis (CMA)	The extra cost was less than that of an alternative programme	Since ΔB is assumed $= 0$, select the programme if $\Delta C < 0$	Focus only on costs	Benefits must be equivalent (i.e., $\Delta B = 0$)

since the money metric is used to measure value in many arenas. The profit maximizing firm described above had all outcomes measured in monetary units and represented in ΔR (which might also be described as a change in benefits, ΔB). Projects where $\Delta B > \Delta C$ are ones in which the extra benefits outweigh the extra costs. Conversely, projects where $\Delta B < \Delta C$ are ones in which the extra benefits are outweighed by the extra costs. The incremental net benefit (INB) is $\Delta B - \Delta C$, which is positive (negative) when extra benefits outweigh (are outweighed by) extra costs. The decision rule in CBA is quite simple: invest in programmes where INB > 0.

It seems appealing to have all measures in monetary units. However, CBA is generally not the first choice of analysts working in the health care field, since there are concerns about placing monetary values on all the consequences of programmes. In contrast, CEA and CUA are more common.

Cost-effectiveness analysis (CEA)

Cost-effectiveness analysis (CEA) has the key outcome measured in natural units. For example, an OHS programme for musculoskeletal disorders in the workplace might focus on reducing absenteeism as a primary objective. A CEA could measure this outcome as days absent from work due to musculoskeletal disorders. Suppose after the introduction of the OHS programme the incremental effect (ΔE) was 100 less absence days and the incremental cost (ΔC) was $32,000. The incremental cost and effect are often combined into a ratio ($\Delta C/\Delta E$) called the incremental cost-effectiveness ratio (ICER). In this case, the ICER = $320 per day of reduced absence due to musculoskeletal disorders. The ICER is an incremental measure and gives different information from that gleaned from simple averages (Hoch and Dewa 2008).

There is usually little controversy about how the outcome is best measured in a CEA, although there may be some concern regarding whether the chosen outcome captured all of the relevant consequences. If this is a concern, different ICERs can be calculated using different outcomes. Calculating multiple ICERs provides an opportunity to compare results using different measures of 'success.' When multiple outcome measures are used, it is possible that conflicting advice may be offered by the ICERs. For example, a disability management programme might decrease absenteeism, but increase presenteeism. Moreover, different outcomes may overlap in terms of the underlying phenomenon that is being measured. For example, presenteeism may capture varying levels of productivity associated with health; a separate measure of productivity may result in double counting. Essentially, it is important to remember that a study's findings regarding the merits of a programme rest upon the measure(s) of effectiveness chosen (Hoch and Dewa 2007).

Forming an opinion about whether the estimated ICER represents good value for money involves making a value judgement. If the decision maker felt a worker absence was worth $350 to prevent, then the OHS programme would, other things equal, be cost-effective. Claiming that something is cost-effective is equivalent to saying that the extra effect is worth the extra cost. In many economic evaluations, the ICER generally indicates that a new treatment is relatively more costly but also relatively more effective than usual care. In these situations, the ICER provides an estimate of the cost and effect trade-off, not a decision about the worthwhileness of the trade-off. Decision makers must determine if INB > 0 based on their willingness to pay for a unit of effect.

Cost–utility analysis (CUA)

When health related utility measures are the outcome of interest, the analysis is called a cost–utility analysis (CUA). Utility values are used to combine reductions in morbidity and extensions of life into a single measure. In health care technology assessments a commonly used outcome measure is the QALY and we shall use it in all our examples of this kind of analysis.

There are various methods of calculating QALYs and there is evidence that there are important differences in their estimates depending on the methods used (Krabbe *et al.* 1997; Gold *et al.* 2002; Arnesen and Trommald 2004; McGregor and Caro 2006). Furthermore, one can get different QALY amounts using the same method depending upon the population that is asked about their values (Shumway 2003). The perspective of the analysis should guide the choice about what population might be most appropriate to sample.

The decision rule using the INB in a CUA can be framed similarly to that for CBA. The INB is now calculated as $\lambda \Delta QALYs - \Delta C$, where λ is the willingness to pay for a QALY. If $\lambda \Delta QALYs - \Delta C > 0$, then the programme represents good value for money. This is because $\Delta B \equiv \lambda \Delta/QALYs$ and if the INB > 0, the value of the incremental benefits outweighs the incremental costs (ΔC). An alternative way to express it is that the extra cost of an extra QALY (i.e., $\Delta C/\Delta QALY$) is less than the decision maker's willingness to pay for an extra QALY (λ).

Cost-minimization analysis (CMA)

In CMA, the only measure of interest is the difference in cost or ΔC. A CMA assesses which choice is cheaper. The choice to use CMA implies that the decision maker is satisfied that the alternatives being considered are sufficiently equivalent in all the important outcomes for the differences not to matter. In the example from Box 9.1, $\Delta C > 0$ for all of the programmes, indicating that all require an investment of funds (we return to this example later to describe the decision making steps). In situations where there may be a difference in effectiveness (i.e. $\Delta E \neq 0$), CMA is inappropriate as it will provide only the cost side of the picture. If the effectiveness of alternatives options is not similar, one should adopt an economic evaluation method that allows competing programmes or interventions to have different levels of effectiveness, such as CBA, CEA or CUA.

Cost–consequence analysis (CCA)

When there are many measures available to represent the effects of a programme, the results can be presented in a cost–consequence analysis (CCA). In CCA costs and consequences are calculated but not combined into a

Box 9.1 Example with hypothetical data to illustrate the decision making steps

Step 1: List cost and effectiveness data for OHS programmes from least to most effective.

Programme	Type	Costs	Effects (QALYs)	ΔCost	ΔEffect	ΔCost / ΔEffect
Low Back Injury	Do nothing	$100,000	1,000			
	Current	$150,000	1,001	$50,000	1	$50,000
	Novel	$160,000	1,002	$10,000	1	$10,000
Repetitive Strain Injury	Bad Idea	$210,000	1,900			
	Do nothing	$200,000	2,000	–$10,000	100	–$100
	Current	$205,000	2,001	$5,000	1	$5,000
	Novel	$225,000	2,002	$20,000	1	$20,000

Step 2: Check for extended dominance after removing dominated options.

Programme	Type	Costs	Effects (QALYs)	ΔCost	ΔEffect	ΔCost / ΔEffect
Low Back Injury	Do nothing	$100,000	1,000			
	Current	$150,000	1,001	$50,000	1	$50,000
	Novel	$160,000	1,002	$10,000	1	$10,000
Repetitive Strain Injury	Do nothing	$200,000	2,000			
	Current	$205,000	2,001	$5,000	1	$5,000
	Novel	$225,000	2,002	$20,000	1	$20,000

Step 3: Calculate relevant decision making ratios.

Programme	Type	Costs	Effects (QALYs)	ΔCost	ΔEffect	ΔCost / ΔEffect
Low Back Injury	Do nothing	$100,000	1,000			
	Novel	$160,000	1,002	$60,000	2	$30,000
Repetitive Strain	Do nothing	$200,000	2,000			
Injury	Current	$205,000	2,001	$5,000	1	$5,000
	Novel	$225,000	2,002	$20,000	1	$20,000

Step 4: Rank by ratio and compare cost to the budget.

Echelon	Programme	Type	Cost ($)	ΔCost / ΔEffect
1	Repetitive Strain Injury	Current	$205,000	$5,000
2		Novel	$225,000	$20,000
3	Low Back Injury	Novel	$160,000	$30,000

With a budget of $205,000, only the programme in Echelon 1 is selected. With a budget of $225,000, only the programme in Echelon 2 is selected. With a budget of $385,000 both programmes in Echelon 2 and 3 are selected.

summary measure. Some feel that this kind of analysis provides the most comprehensive presentation of information describing the value of a programme or intervention, and is also conceptually the simplest (Mauskopf *et al.* 1998), although it leaves much of the trading-off to be done 'in committee' by decision makers unless the analyst combines all effects into a composite summary measure.

Decision rules for cost-effectiveness and cost–utility analysis

In the discussion that follows we will assume the choices are all or nothing and set aside matters of the scale and intensity of possible interventions. This enables us to focus on trade-offs and how they fit into optimal decisions. For a more technical treatment see Weinstein and Zeckhauser (1973), together with the reaction of Birch and Gafni (1992), and the response to the reaction by Johannesson and Weinstein (1993). An attempt at a resolution of the earlier feud is made by Stinnett and Paltiel (1996). Other attempts to guide resource allocation decision making using economic evaluation include Garber and Phelps (1997).

Quantifying trade-offs helps to answer two fundamental questions. The first relates to whether a programme should be adopted at all. The answer to this is: invest if the extra benefit is at least as great as the extra cost (i.e., $\Delta B \geq \Delta C$). The second question relates to how much OHS to invest in (or how many programmes to adopt). Here, the answer is to invest in OHS to the point where the extra benefit equals the extra cost. For example, if $\Delta B > \Delta C$, then more should be invested. Conversely, if $\Delta B < \Delta C$, then less should be invested (see Figure 9.1 and 9.2 for illustrations of these concepts).

Before making a decision about which programmes to fund, it is first necessary to sort programmes into groups based on the OHS issue addressed by each programme, and then list them by increasing effectiveness within each group. Grouping alternatives in this way allows one to consider how attractive each option is compared with alternatives addressing the same health and safety concerns. For example, assume that a decision maker is considering two types of novel OHS programmes. One is for primary prevention of low back injury and another is for primary prevention of repetitive strain injury (RSI). Box 9.1 elaborates on this example [readers interested in a more detailed example involving extended dominance and many programmes are referred to Karlsson and Johannesson (1996)].

Assume that the novel low back injury programme costs $160,000 and the novel RSI programme $225,000. Each produces two extra QALYs compared with the 'do-nothing' alternative. Of primary interest is the extra cost (ΔC)

and the extra effect (ΔE) generated by these programmes compared with the next most effective alternative (see Step 1 in Box 9.1). Three options exist for low back injury: the novel programme, the current programme, and doing nothing.

Four options exist for RSI: the novel programme, the current programme, doing nothing, and a 'bad idea'. The ΔC and the ΔE are computed relative to the next most effective programme option, which is why the programmes should be sorted by increasing effectiveness. Typically, the ratio of ΔC to ΔE (i.e., the ICER) is calculated as an estimate of the extra cost for an extra unit of effect. Once the ΔCs and ΔEs have been calculated, the proposed programmes can be selected using three additional steps (see Steps 2–4 in Box 9.1).

Step 2 involves reviewing the programme alternatives to remove dominated (economically irrelevant) programmes. If a less effective programme has higher costs than its more effective comparator, it should be dropped from further consideration. The more effective programme is said to dominate because it is better in terms of both cost and effect (this is known as 'strong dominance'). An example is the 'bad idea' to treat RSI. It is both more expensive and less effective than doing nothing. As a result, it is discarded from the decision-making process in Step 2 because of strong dominance.

Weak dominance occurs when a comparator is better in either the cost or the effect category (but equivalent in the other). If the 'bad idea' for the RSI yielded 2,000 QALYs (instead of 1,900 QALYs), it would still be weakly dominated by doing nothing, which would be as effective, but less costly. In any case, all dominated programmes should be removed before the economic data are used to prioritize programmes by efficiency, so that only relevant programmes are considered.

If programmes can be resized without affecting the relationship between costs and effects, it is essential to check for programmes that could be ruled out because of extended dominance. Extended dominance can be detected by using the $\Delta C/\Delta E$ ratios, after removing strongly and weakly dominated programmes. If a less effective programme has a larger $\Delta C/\Delta E$ ratio than the next more effective programme, this indicates extended dominance in a set of mutually exclusive programmes. For example, in Step 2 in Box 9.1, the first $\Delta C/\Delta E$ ratio in the low back injury category is $50,000 per extra QALY and the next $\Delta C/\Delta E$ ratio in that category is $10,000 per extra QALY. There is extended dominance since the less effective programme has a higher ICER ($50,000 per QALY) than the next more effective programme ($10,000 per QALY). A combination of doing nothing and investing in the novel programme would be better than doing the current programme. Specifically, if the novel programme was used 5/6th of the time and doing nothing 1/6th of the time, this combination would cost $150,000 for 1,001.67 QALYs ($160,000 × 5/6 + $100,000 × 1/6 = $150,000;

and 1,002 QALYs × 5/6 + 1,000 QALYs × 1/6 = 1,001.67 QALYs). Hence, the cost is $150,000 both for the combined strategy and the current programme, so $\Delta C = 0$. However, the combination option is more effective than the current programme ($\Delta E = 0.67$).

All programmes that are dominated (whether strongly, weakly, or by extension) should be removed, and the $\Delta C/\Delta E$ ratios then recalculated (see Step 3 in Box 9.1). The recalculation is necessary since any removal of programmes could change the ΔC and ΔE for those that remain.

Lastly, programmes ought to be listed in order of least to most expensive in terms of cost per additional unit of effect (see Step 4 in Box 9.1). As noted by Johannesson (1995), the ordering of the ratios of mutually exclusive programmes cannot be interpreted as a ranking list, since only one can be implemented, and the choice depends on the size of the budget.

What is the decision maker's willingness to pay for the additional outcome? Because λ is typically unknown, a frequently adopted strategy in applied work is to assume a value for λ and then suggest investing in all programmes having a $\Delta C/\Delta E$ ratio less than λ. For example, based on $\lambda = \$60,000$ per QALY, one economic evaluation of an OHS programme for clinicians recommended selective vaccination for physicians and for paramedical workers, since ICERs for both were less than $60,000 (Chodick *et al.* 2002).

Alternatively, programmes can be selected based on the $\Delta C/\Delta E$ ratio and the size of the budget. Here, we assume the decision maker seeks to maximize outcomes subject to a budget constraint, and will spend all of the budget, but no more. For example, with a budget of $205,000, only the current RSI programme (at $5,000 per QALY) could be funded (since even if the decision maker felt that $60,000 was a reasonable amount to pay for an extra QALY, with a binding budget constraint there is no more money to be spent). With a budget of $225,000, only the novel RSI programme would be selected. With a budget of $385,000 both the novel RSI and lower back injury programmes would be selected.

Dealing with the uncertainty about the value of λ

After reporting the results of an economic evaluation, the analysis may follow with an assessment of whether the trade-off of ΔC for ΔE is worthwhile (i.e., whether the programme or intervention is cost-effective). If we knew the λ for an additional QALY or any additional desirable outcome, then we could compare it to our ICER price tag.

The analysis of the worthwhileness of the trade-off might be aided by appealing to previous decisions. For example, if decision makers typically selected programmes that were around $50,000 per additional QALY, then perhaps they would fund a new OHS programme with an ICER of $50,000 per QALY. While precedent may help to provide context, it has been argued that decisions made in this way can lead to uncontrolled growth in expenditures (Birch and Gafni 1992; Gafni and Birch 2003).

In practice it is likely that there will be considerable uncertainty surrounding the willingness to pay for an additional unit of outcome. Sensitivity analysis can be used to see how the INB changes with different values of λ (e.g., Hoch *et al.* 2002; Hoch and Smith 2006). Given that the INB estimate is accompanied by statistical uncertainty, a cost-effectiveness acceptability curve (CEAC) is often used to summarize the results of a CEA or CUA (Briggs and Fenn 1998; Löthgren and Zethraeus 2000; Fenwick *et al.* 2001,2006; Hoch *et al.* 2006). A CEAC highlights the relationship between the probability of cost-effectiveness and the unknown λ (see Figure 9.3 for an example).

The shape of the CEAC identifies how sensitive the probability of cost-effectiveness is to assumptions about λ. For example, the figure in Figure 9.3 shows that when λ is within a $500 range of the ICER estimate (i.e. $596– $1,596) the probability of cost-effectiveness is quite sensitive to the value chosen for λ. If λ = $500, the probability of the OHS programme being cost-effective is 0%, but at λ = $1,500 it is approximately 88%. Most of the dramatic gains in the height of the CEAC (from 0 to 88%) occur between λ = $500 and $1,500. Alternatively, the curve is mostly flat for λ < $500 and λ > $1,500. While the real value of λ may be unknown, if it is assumed to be more than $1,500, it is, in this example, highly probable that the OHS programme is cost-effective.

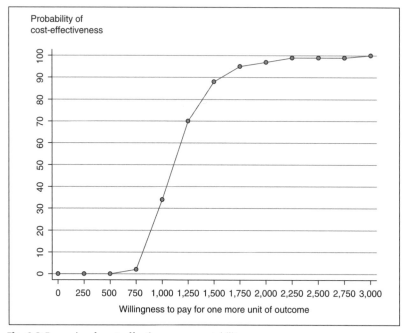

Fig. 9.3 Example of cost-effectiveness acceptability curve.

Recommendations

Perhaps the most important advice to be drawn from this chapter is the importance of being transparent about the reason for selecting a particular kind of economic analysis, the outcome of focus, and the accompanying decision rule. Our recommendations are as follows:

- Use one or more appropriate comparator(s) in an economic evaluation and be explicit about what they are. Without a comparator, the ΔC and ΔB (or ΔE) cannot be computed. When the appropriate comparator really has no cost and no effect, then the $\Delta C/\Delta E$ ratio reduces to C/E. In this case the C/E ratio is really an ICER, but the comparison scenario has $C = E = 0$.

- For CBA, use the efficiency decision rule: 'adopt interventions having a positive incremental net-present value' (i.e., $\Delta B - \Delta C > 0$).

- For CEA and CUA, use the efficiency decision rule: 'adopt interventions where the extra cost is less than the value of the extra outcome (i.e. $\lambda \Delta E - \Delta C > 0$).'

- Ensure that the choice of the kind of economic evaluation reflects what the decision maker feels is of most importance in terms of outcomes and her/his objectives for the programme. For example, while the QALY is widely used in the health care field, it may not always be as meaningful in OHS interventions.

- Do not assume that the efficiency decision rules are dominant over other considerations, such as the equity of the distribution of costs and consequences, and the feasibility of implementation.

- Be clear about the perspective from which the study is to be done and the level of decision making (e.g., firm, system, societal).

- Be transparent about areas of uncertainty and assumptions, so that the decision maker can place results in her/his own context. For example, an OHS programme with an economically attractive ICER could be too costly for a decision maker.

- Indicate key data that are judged to have been measured well and those measured poorly. Avoid combining both types into a single number.

- Consider trade-offs when presenting options and focus on the opportunity costs (e.g., what would be forgone in order to pay for the current candidate programme).

- Compare results with those of other similar studies where these exist.

- Explicitly consider the issues raised for regulation and/or subsidy when societal considerations indicate the net desirability of an intervention, but the organization sees only net costs.

Appendix 1: derivation of optimal solution with $\Delta R = \Delta C$

Assume a profit maximizing firm must purchase labour (L) at wage rate w, capital (K) at rate r, and occupational health and safety (OHS) services at rate p_{OHS}. Thus, the firm's cost equation is:

$$\text{Cost} = wL + rK + p_{OHS}\text{OHS}. \qquad [A1.1]$$

The firm sells its output (Q) at price (p). Thus, the firm's revenue equation is:

$$\text{Revenue} = pQ. \qquad [A1.2]$$

The concept of a full time equivalent (FTE) is used to introduce the idea that workers may not always be in perfect health. The variable 'health' is defined on a scale from 0 to 1, such that 10 workers each with health = 0.5, can do the work of five healthy workers. Thus, the firm's production function is:

$$Q = f(FTE, K), \qquad [A1.3]$$

where

$$FTE = g(L, \text{health}) = L \times \text{health} \qquad [A1.4]$$

and

$$\text{health} = h(\text{OHS}; Z), \qquad [A1.5]$$

where Z is a set of exogenous factors. The for-profit firm chooses L, K and OHS to maximize:

$$\pi = pQ - \text{Cost}, \qquad [A1.6]$$
$$\pi = p \times f(\text{FTE}, K) - wL - rK - p_{OHS}\text{OHS}, \qquad [A1.7]$$
$$\pi = p \times f\{[L \times \text{health}(\text{OHS}; Z)], K\} - wL - rK - p_{OHS}\text{OHS}, \qquad [A1.8]$$

since

$$Q = f\{FTE[L, \text{health}(\text{OHS}; Z)], K\} = f\{[L \times \text{health}(\text{OHS}; Z)], K\}.$$

To illustrate the reasoning behind decision rules in the text, the partial derivative of [A1.8] is taken with respect to OHS:

$$\partial\pi/\partial\text{OHS} = p(\partial f/\partial FTE)(\partial FTE/\partial\text{health})(\partial\text{health}/\partial\text{OHS}) - p_{OHS} = 0.$$
$$p(\partial f/\partial FTE)(\partial FTE/\partial\text{health})(\partial\text{health}/\partial\text{OHS}) = p_{OHS}.$$
since $p(\partial FTE/(\partial\text{health}) = pL$
then

$$pL(\partial f/(\text{FTE})(\partial \text{health}/\partial \text{OHS}) = p_{\text{OHS}}.$$

The interpretation of this last expression is:

(value of marginal product FTE)(marginal improvement in health)

= (marginal cost of OHS).

So, $\partial \pi/\partial \text{OHS} = 0$ when the marginal revenue equals the marginal cost of OHS.

Appendix 2: derivation of optimal solution of constrained optimization

Assume a decision maker is concerned with both reducing morbidity and extending life for a population. To operationalize this goal, we assume the relevant objective is to maximize quality adjusted life years (QALYs). QALYs are assumed to be a function of the quantity of the occupational health and safety (OHS) interventions and other programmes (OTHER) that the decision maker funds. The provision/purchase of programmes is limited because of a budget constraint. We assume the budget constraint is exogenous, and is of the form:

$$Y = P_{\text{OHS}}\text{OHS} + P_{\text{OTHER}}\text{OTHER}, \qquad [\text{A2.1}]$$

where Y is the total budget, P_{OHS} and P_{OTHER} are the unit prices for OHS and OTHER, respectively. Thus, when the entire budget is spent on OHS, an amount equal to Y/P_{OHS} can be purchased. The best way for a decision maker to spend the money is related to the objective, which is assumed to be:

$$\text{Maximize QALYs} = f(\text{OHS, OTHER}), \qquad [\text{A2.2}]$$

where $f()$ is a function that converts OHS and OTHER investments into QALYs. The constrained optimization problem is solved using a Lagrange function:

$$\Lambda = \text{QALYs} + \mu(Y - P_{\text{OHS}}\text{OHS} - P_{\text{OTHER}}\text{OTHER}), \qquad [\text{A2.3}]$$

where μ is the Lagrange multiplier or the shadow price of a dollar in terms of QALYs. Later, we introduce $\lambda = 1/\mu$ as the willingness to pay for an additional QALY. To solve [A2.3], we compute the first order conditions:

$$\partial \Lambda/\partial \text{OHS} = \partial \text{QALY}/\partial \text{OHS} - \mu\, P_{\text{OHS}} = 0, \qquad [\text{A2.4}]$$

$$\partial \Lambda/\partial \text{OTHER} = \partial \text{QALY}/\partial \text{OTHER} - \mu\, P_{\text{OTHER}} = 0, \qquad [\text{A2.5}]$$

$$\partial\Lambda/\partial\mu = Y - P_{OHS}OHS - P_{OTHER}OTHER = 0. \qquad [A2.6]$$

From these equations, a necessary condition for the optimal amount of OHS and OTHER is:

$$(\partial QALY/\partial OHS)/P_{OHS} = (\partial QALY/\partial OTHER)/P_{OTHER} = \mu.$$

Alternatively, we can write this condition as:

ΔCost OHS/ΔQALYs from OHS = ΔCost of OTHER/ΔQALYs from OTHER = λ.

Chapter 10

Costs

Audrey Laporte, Roman Dolinschi, and
Emile Tompa

Introduction

This chapter suggests some good practice procedures in the assessment of the
costs of an intervention. We intend it to be applicable to the entire range
of types of economic evaluation studies—cost–benefit analysis (CBA), cost-
effectiveness analysis (CEA), cost–utility analysis (CUA), cost-minimizing
analysis (CMA), and cost–consequence analysis (CCA)—but caution will have
to be exercised in each context. Economic costs are not immutable entities
that can be easily identified by the inspection of accounts. As has been
explained earlier (see Chapter 2) the underlying idea of a cost is that it is
a monetary sum representing the most valued alternative use of a resource
(i.e., the opportunity cost). Costs will always be contingent on the perspective
of a study and on the nature of the decision [classic references are Alchian
(1959, 1968)]. For example, what appears as a cost in a study from the perspective of a workers' compensation board might be a transfer from a societal
perspective; what is not considered a cost in a study examining only the short-
term consequences of a possible decision may be a cost in a similar study
taking a long-term view. Maintenance costs will be a significant cost component in a decision to introduce and maintain an item of equipment, but not in
a decision to acquire it and sell it shortly thereafter. A decision to implement
an occupational health and safety (OHS) intervention will invariably embody
decisions about the timing (sooner versus later) and the speed (faster versus
slower) of its introduction. Both typically affect costs: generally, the sooner the
implementation the greater the cost; the faster the implementation the greater
the cost. What is always true, however, is that the costs to be considered are the
resource used as a result of the decision in question.

Sometimes there is arbitrariness in the way in which costs are treated in an economic evaluation. For example, it is sometimes suggested that an intervention
whose consequence is longer life for the beneficiaries ought to include the costs
of future health care due to unrelated health problems which the lengthened

life makes likely. There remains some uncertainty amongst economists as to whether such costs are to be legitimately included. However, since such costs are the costs of future decisions (which may not be taken), they are not properly to be considered as costs of the current decision, even though the possibility of the choice which may give rise to them is undoubtedly a consequence of the current decision.

Another source of confusion relates to what are often termed 'indirect costs' (the term 'indirect consequences' or 'indirect benefits' is also used by some). There is less than complete agreement about what constitutes direct versus indirect and we suggest that, rather than labelling costs as indirect, simply identifying them explicitly by name. Our suggested approach is to treat indirect costs as the predictable resources used due to a decision even if they are not the resources directly consumed by the intervention itself (see Box 10.1 for definitions).

The term 'indirect costs' often refers to external costs (i.e., costs that fall on individuals and others that are not party to the decision) and to changes in

---

Box 10.1 Costs and consequences

Indirect costs: the costs incurred by a decision maker and other stakeholders that are not the immediate cost of inputs in the intervention. In particular, the negative impact that an intervention may have on productivity.

Social costs of an OHS intervention: the value of all resources used as a direct consequence of a decision to introduce, execute, and maintain an OHS intervention, regardless on whoever they may fall.

Private costs of an OHS intervention: generally, the expenses incurred by a decision maker, such as the firm, to introduce, execute, and maintain an OHS intervention.

Consequences of an OHS intervention: all changes in health states attributable to an intervention, as well as other values created and resources saved. Values created can include productivity improvements directly due to the intervention and/or mediated through health. Resources saved can include reduced operating costs in several areas within an organization, as well as reduced costs experienced by workers (e.g., as reduced out-of-pocket expenditures for health care) and other stakeholders.

productivity due to the decision. Two types of productivity changes should be distinguished: short-term productivity effects attributable to down time while new equipment is installed and time spent learning to use a new machine or to undertake a new process, and long-term productivity effects directly related to the intervention or mediated through health improvements.

The former are legitimate costs of deciding to execute an intervention, while the latter are consequences of the intervention and may be positive or negative. If they are negative, it is tempting to regard them as costs, whereas it is better to count them as consequences (ones whose value ought to be deducted from the positive benefits). A similar treatment is appropriate when an intervention has the effect of reducing future costs for other reasons. Again, these are not costs of the decision, but (positive) monetary benefits to be counted amongst the other benefits (see Chapter 11 for treatment of productivity consequences, and other values created and resources saved). Our recommendation is that input resources specific to the intervention be treated as costs and all other resource implications be classified as consequences (some might also use the term 'effects' or 'benefits' for consequences).

In most cases, such as a CBA in which an incremental net present value (NPV) of costs and consequences is calculated, the distinction between direct and indirect costs will not be important as long as changes are captured with the correct sign in the summary measure (positive for incremental costs and productivity reductions, and negative for productivity increases). They do matter, however, in the calculation of ratios of costs and consequences, as in CBA, CEA and CUA ratios. It is important when comparing such ratios across different possible investments to make sure that costs and consequences of these types are consistently treated (i.e., included in the numerator or denominator), so as to avoid bias. For CBA, we recommend using the incremental NPV approach, rather than calculating a ratio in order to avoid confusion. For CEA and CUA, all monetary measures are included in the numerator, with only non-monetary measures of health in the denominator.

With respect to perspective, our recommended practice is to select the relevant perspective(s), which is often that of the firm in the case of OHS interventions, as well as a broader (possibly societal) perspective. The relevant perspective(s) should be discussed with stakeholders. Note that even the perspective of the firm can vary. For example, it may include all stakeholders in the firm such as workers, management and owners, or may include only the owner of the firm. In most cases it is taken as the latter.

The inclusion of a broader perspective is recommended in order to determine whether an intervention is of benefit once the full range of costs and consequences is taken into consideration. A broad perspective will help determine if, at the margin (i.e., compared with the alternative), the social costs are less than the consequences experienced by all stakeholders, rather than simply the private costs being less than the consequences experienced by the firm owners. It can also bring to light the distributional implications of options. Excluding particular stakeholders from the analysis may result in a recommendation for an inefficient and inequitable allocation of income and resources across all the affected stakeholders in a jurisdiction. For example, the costs associated with the introduction of an OHS intervention may reside primarily with the owners of a firm though the benefits accruing to it may be small, whereas the benefits accruing to workers and their families may be substantial and their costs small. If the firm perspective is the only one taken in an evaluation, the intervention might appear not to be worthwhile, yet from a broader perspective it may indeed be worth undertaking (the reverse may also be the case). Exclusion of a broad perspective may also generate resentment amongst groups whose co-operation is crucial for the successful implementation of the intervention. To assess societal level efficiency issues, as well as the distributional impact of alternatives, costs and consequences should be considered at the aggregate level as well as on a disaggregated basis by stakeholder and cost category.

Taking a broad perspective is particularly important in OHS because of the range of stakeholders typically involved and the possible inter-relationship between programmes and funding. Key stakeholders to consider include: firm owners, the public sector (e.g., ministries with OHS legislative, inspection oversight and service provision responsibilities) and insurance providers (e.g., health care insurers, short-term and long-term disability insurance providers, other public pensions), and workers and their families.

Figure 10.1 identifies some possible costs and consequences associated with an OHS intervention and the stakeholders to which they might accrue. This is by no means a comprehensive list of costs, consequences, and stakeholders affected, but it is a summary of the ones generally considered as most relevant for OHS interventions. To identify the full complement of stakeholders affected by an intervention, it is useful to consider the organisational structure of the OHS system in question (see Chapter 6).

Identification and treatment of costs

An economic evaluation requires the comparison of two or more relevant alternatives. The comparator is often the status quo or standard OHS practices in existence prior to the introduction of an intervention. Regardless of the

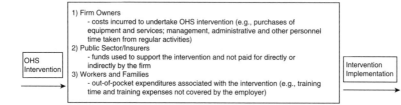

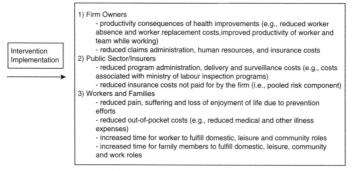

Fig. 10.1 Categories of OHS intervention costs and consequences.

comparator, the focus is on incremental costs (and incremental consequences), rather than on total costs (and total consequences). We assume that the status quo is the usual comparator in our discussion of costs, but our suggestions for good practice apply to comparisons with one or more alternative interventions.

Costs can be subdivided into several categories: capital expenditure/equipment purchase or upgrade costs, expenses for external intervention facilitators and consultants, time devoted to intervention by firm's management and human resource department, worker time devoted to intervention, and miscellaneous costs.

The firm's formal or informal equipment replacement and upgrade policy will be an important factor to consider in identifying incremental costs associated with capital expenditures and equipment purchases. Only the incremental costs of new or upgraded equipment, such as ergonomically more advanced chairs or keyboards, should be attributed to the intervention since the expense of standard equipment would have been incurred even if the intervention was not introduced. (See Box 10.2 for an example of a study that takes this into consideration). If firms do not have formal procedures and timelines for equipment upgrading or replacement, information on informal policies and practices can be elicited from interviews with their management.

Key factors in assessing cost flows for equipment are: the expected lifetime of new equipment, the rate of (annual) depreciation, and expenses associated with maintenance such as service contracts.

Since the remaining years of usefulness of equipment decrease over time, this depreciation should be reflected in the assessment of cost flows. Within the cost flows, it is also necessary to account for any expenses associated with maintenance.

Costs related to hiring intervention facilitators or consultants, such as ergonomic experts, can be significant. All service fees and time costs of the experts associated with the intervention, which can include provision of expertise and guidance during the implementation stage, training time, purchase of training materials, and so on, need to be included. Anticipated future charges associated with expert services (i.e., consultant fees and costs to administer retraining of existing or new staff) should also be included if they are associated with maintenance of the intervention planned to be in place for an extended period of time.

Box 10.2 A study that considered a company's equipment replacement policy

Lanoie and Tavenas (1996) investigated the introduction of a participatory ergonomics intervention at an alcohol products distribution warehouse in Quebec, Canada. The researchers consulted the company's equipment replacement policy to identify incremental equipment costs attributable to the additional features deemed necessary for the intervention by the joint working committee. As a result, when new trucks were purchased by the warehouse, only the cost of ergonomic seats was included in the analysis as the trucks were due for replacement anyway. The researchers also considered costs related to the extra time required to operate a new packaging machine. Projections of future costs (accounting for expected inflation) were made that included future maintenance expenses associated with the new equipment and purchases of necessary materials.

Researchers may sometimes play dual roles as both facilitators or consultants and intervention evaluators. Costs associated with evaluating the intervention should not be included, as these are research costs not inherent in the decision unless the evaluation is a condition of implementation. Researchers who also serve as consultants will need to document time spent in one role versus the other so that consultant time can be separated from evaluation time.

Regarding human resources personnel and management time, the key is to capture the incremental cost of time spent by these individuals on the new OHS activities relative to the pre-intervention status quo. Researchers need to examine whether and to what extent the OHS function is a part of management's and human resources department's standard responsibility. If the intervention adds substantially to their time spent on OHS activities, resulting either in overtime hours or in hours being diverted from other activities, the value of this additional time is part of the intervention cost. The relevant wage rates, including benefits, are generally used to value this time. Larger firms are more likely to have dedicated in-house OHS staff or managers who are able to direct their time toward such activities, compared with smaller firms. Thus, in larger firms, incremental management and human resources personnel time costs are likely to be relatively small.

Workers may be taken away from regular production activities for a variety of reasons associated with the intervention. There may be down time due to equipment replacement or installation and time will be spent being trained on the use of new equipment and/or new OHS policies and practices. Furthermore, the firm may incur costs of replacing workers, while core staff are being trained. Such up-front and future time costs of worker involvement in the intervention should be accounted for in the analysis.

Not all costs of worker time associated with the intervention are incurred by the employer (e.g., unpaid hours spent in training by workers outside of work hours). Personal worker time costs may be incurred at various points throughout the intervention time frame and should be included if a broad (societal) perspective is taken. As with manager's time, worker time can be valued using the worker's hourly wage rate, including benefits.

There may be other costs associated with an intervention that do not fall into any of the above categories. These may be easily quantifiable such as travel expenses to an external training facility or not so easily quantifiable, such as team production losses due to disruption during the introduction of the intervention. Where possible, such costs should be measured and included in the analysis, or at the minimum commented on in the text of the evaluation.

Applicable sales taxes should be included if the perspective being considered is that of the firm. From a societal perspective sales taxes are simply transfers, so they would be excluded. In presenting disaggregated costs, taxes are an expense for the firm, but an equivalent gain (ignoring transaction costs) in the form of tax receipts for the public sector.

All cost flows should be identified by the year they occur, adjusted for inflation using a price index, and discounted to the year the intervention is to begin (see Chapter 12 for details).

Data sources

A firm's administrative records are a valuable source of data for estimating intervention costs. In-house sources include: payroll records of wages, salaries, and benefits of workers and managers, and hours worked; human resource policies; and other policies, such as an equipment replacement and upgrade policy.

Administrative records can also provide data for evaluating consequences (e.g., data on health outcomes, such as first aid incidents, modified duty episodes, casual absenteeism, workers' compensation claims, or private insurance claims).

A management survey might be used to gather detailed information on the distribution of OHS responsibilities across managers, the processes affected by the intervention, the relevant cost categories to consider, and the policies and practices affecting costs associated with the intervention. Some examples of information that might be collected in a survey include: the amount of time generally spent by managers on OHS issues and the additional hours spent to facilitate the intervention; details of production time lost by workers due to involvement in the intervention, and the staff reallocation undertaken to accommodate this; details of the standard expenses incurred for equipment, materials and service and the incremental ones associated with the intervention; details of external consultant services; and other costs associated with the intervention that may not be immediately evident to the researchers, including anticipated future costs.

A worker survey might be used to supplement a management survey. It can be used to provide details about the number of paid hours absent from production activities due to the intervention (e.g. idle time during workstation redesign, time spent on training, and time spent on intervention committees), the number of unpaid hours devoted to intervention activities, and estimates of the number of hours workers anticipate spending on future intervention-related activities.

To minimize the research costs of the study and to ensure access to the most suitable cost data, researchers should design the mechanisms to be used to collect data for the economic part of an evaluation in conjunction with other study design elements and collect relevant data at the same time as data is collected for the effectiveness evaluation (for a detailed discussion of issues related to data sources see Chapter 7).

Issues related to the treatment of costs

Accurate valuation of costs can present unanticipated critical challenges. Four issues in particular stand out: measurement of changes at the margin; distinguishing transfers, market prices, and opportunity costs; the treatment of future costs; and accounting for the human resource structure of a firm or industry. We consider each of these in turn, with a focus on the firm and societal perspectives.

Measurement of changes at the margin

It is incremental or marginal changes, rather than absolute or total amounts that usually matter because the intent of an economic evaluation is to focus on the differences between options. In other words, what is relevant is not the total cost and total benefit of an OHS intervention, but the incremental costs (marginal cost) and incremental benefits (marginal benefit) associated with one option relative to another, often the status quo. If the marginal cost is less than the marginal benefit (and the desirable consequences are the same or greater), then the intervention is worth undertaking, since it will increase firm profits, efficiency in the OHS system, or social welfare, depending on the perspective taken. Thus, it is only costs over and above the alternative, or those normally incurred if the alternative is the status quo, that are of interest and likewise it is only the difference in consequences that needs to be calculated (see Chapter 9 on kind of analysis for details). A common error in many published economic evaluations of OHS interventions is attributing all new costs incurred during the intervention period, rather than the incremental costs, to the intervention under investigation.

Transfer prices, market prices, and opportunity costs

Inaccurate measurement of costs may arise when prices are generated within a firm for accounting purposes to allow for transfers and billing between departments. This can also be the case for transfers between government departments. For example, a manufacturer may produce door handles and doors. The firm could sell the door handles to other manufacturers and the public, or it can install them in the doors they also manufacture. In the latter case, simply using the transfer price of the door handles would not necessarily reflect the market value or opportunity cost of that output. Yet, if an analyst is evaluating an intervention that prevents injuries amongst workers in the door handle production department, the market price of production should be considered. If transfer prices do not reflect true market prices, the analyst can look to the market to identify costs for similar products or services. Essentially, the opportunity cost relevant to the perspective taken should be considered.

The market price can be an inaccurate measure of value if a competitive market does not exist for a good or service. For example, if a premium is paid for a good or service such as specialty clinician services and new pharmaceutical products due to restricted entry to that market, the market price (even after allowing for overheads such as research costs) may exaggerate the opportunity cost at the societal level. If a societal perspective is taken, an adjustment needs to be made to the market price, for example by using the prices of comparable products and services. If a firm perspective is taken, the actual purchase cost incurred by the firm would be the relevant price to use in an analysis. Essentially, the opportunity cost can vary for the same good or service depending on the perspective.

In summary, some prices are likely to reflect things such as accounting conventions, tax laws, or premiums due to restricted market entry, and therefore give a distorted picture of true opportunity cost, whether they are prices distorted by taxes and monopoly pricing, and whether the analysis is being conducted from a societal perspective or from the narrower one of the firm or division within a firm. The analyst must accordingly take care to ensure that prices used in the analysis reflect the true resource implications to the decision maker.

Treatment of future costs and consequences

The inclusion of unmeasured future costs and consequences (i.e., those that extend beyond the measurement time frame) is a highly debated issue (Drummond and Sculpher 2005). In many cases substantial costs and consequences may occur in the future, and failure to take longer-term cost effects into account can bias a study in either direction. Box 10.3 provides an example of an evaluation study that considered both the measurement time frame (the stop-and-drop approach) and projections into the future. Most studies take the conservative stop-and-drop approach in which no costs or consequences are considered after the measurement time period. However, this conservatism does not imply that the direction of bias is known (for example, it does not imply that truncating the data in this way means that costs will always be underestimated or overestimated relative to consequences).

Box 10.3 Stop-and-drop approach versus projections of future costs and consequences

The study described in Box 10.2 (Lanoie and Tavenas 1996) considered two time frames. It provides a good example of how consideration of future costs and consequences can substantially change the findings of an evaluation.

The first time frame considered in the evaluation was the measurement time frame (the stop-and-drop approach). The second time frame was an analytic time frame of 10 years. The researchers found that the participatory ergonomics intervention being evaluated in the study was financially rewarding for the firm only in the second scenario. One shortcoming of the second time frame analysis is that the researchers did not test the robustness of their finding to the assumptions underlying their projection of future costs and consequences, although a sensitivity analysis was performed on the discount rate.

Statistical modelling has become increasingly the answer to estimating future costs and consequences in the pharmaco-economic literature, though both the specification and estimation of models poses challenges and is not without controversy. Failing to model longer-term effects is not, of course, a response that resolves the problem of bias. The validity of estimates of effects derived from models rests primarily on the quality of the data that they are drawn from and the credibility of the model into which they are incorporated. A sensitivity analysis should always be undertaken to assess the robustness of findings to the assumptions underlying the model and the possible ranges of the estimates derived from it (see Chapter 12 for details). We recommend supplementing the stop-and-drop approach whenever possible by using modelled projections into the future, along with sensitivity analyses of the key underlying assumptions built into the projections (see Box 10.3).

Human resource structure of the firm and industry

Employment relationships between workers and employers vary widely. Workers can be full-time or part-time, permanent or temporary/casual, unionized or non-unionized, or the work may be done by an independent contractor or another firm. In some jurisdictions, workers who are independent contractors are not covered by workers' compensation insurance. The nature of the employment relationships will affect the incidence of injury costs and the benefits of prevention efforts. Some firms may be better able to externalize risk (and costs) by hiring temporary workers, independent contractors, or by outsourcing work to other firms. Consideration of the types of employer–worker/service provider relationships and the characteristics of the firm (e.g. large or small, unionized or non-unionized) is important to assessing the distribution of costs and consequences. From the firm perspective, only costs incurred by the firm should be included in the analysis, and these may vary depending on the nature of the employment/service contract (all the more reason for the analyst to consider a broad perspective). From the societal perspective, the full cost of all labour time should be used.

Recommendations

In summary, our recommendations pertaining to the treatment of costs in an economic evaluation are as follows:

- Make the analytic and measurement time frame explicit.
- Ensure that costs are reasonable approximations to opportunity costs, given the perspective.
- Use incremental rather than total or average costs.
- Consider the decision context (e.g., timing and speed of introduction, and duration of the intervention) and the ways in which that might affect costs.
- Consider including costs of the intervention occurring beyond the measurement time frame and be explicit about how they are formulated.
- For CBA, add together with the appropriate sign incremental costs and consequences (negative for costs, positive for positive monetary consequences, and negative for negative monetary consequences) to determine the incremental net present value.
- For CEA or CUA, place incremental monetary costs and consequences in the numerator with positive consequences subtracted from costs and negative consequences added to costs.
- Distinguish, in the detailed reporting, between productivity costs (inputs to the intervention such as worker time for training and down time for new equipment installation) and productivity consequences (e.g., increases in productivity and/or product quality directly due to the intervention or mediated through health).
- Present disaggregated costs by component and stakeholder in addition to a summary measure.
- Present time losses and wage rates separately.

- Adjust costs for inflation so that all estimates are in constant prices (see Chapter 12 for details).

- Discount costs using an appropriate discount rate (see Chapter 12 for details).

- Test the impact of various assumptions about costs through sensitivity analysis (see Chapter 12 for details).

Chapter 11

Consequences

Emile Tompa, Roman Dolinschi, and
Claire de Oliveira

Introduction

This chapter is about measuring the consequences of occupational health
and safety (OHS) interventions. Consequences include changes in health
states, as well as non-health values created and resources saved. Improvements
in health or reductions in its rate of deterioration, are the most important
outcome of interest in OHS. Health is of value to individuals for several
reasons; it is of value for its own sake and also because it makes other things
possible. Good health facilitates the fulfilment of social roles, such as working,
domestic responsibilities, parenting, undertaking community service,
and enjoying leisure. Reductions in work disability and their related productivity implications are central to OHS interventions. These are attained
through interventions directed at primary, secondary, and tertiary prevention
(see Box 11.1 for definitions). Other important values created and resources
saved due to OHS interventions include reduced claims administration
expenses, reduced health care expenditures and reduced out-of-pocket
expenses for workers.

Most evaluations of OHS interventions compare a new intervention to
the status quo or the standard practice, but the comparator can also be an
alternative intervention or there could be several comparators. In some OHS
studies, the comparator is not explicitly stated, but is implicitly the status quo
prior to the new intervention. The practice of not explicitly stating the
comparator is not recommended, but is common in many OHS studies.
In this chapter, we shall assume that the comparator is the status quo unless
otherwise stated, although the principles outlined are equally applicable to
other comparators.

Most economic evaluations of OHS interventions implicitly or explicitly
take the firm owner's perspective. However, there is a strong normative argument for considering and adopting a broader perspective. The fact that many
stakeholders can be affected by OHS issues (e.g., firm owner(s), insurer(s),

Box 11.1 Types of prevention

Primary prevention: activities designed to reduce the occurrence of new cases of injury and disease, such as the purchase of safer equipment to reduce risk exposures.

Secondary prevention: activities targeted at reducing the duration of existing injuries and diseases through, for example, early reporting and treatment.

Tertiary prevention: activities designed to reduce the impact of established injuries and diseases on social roles, such as work, by restoring functional ability or role performance through accommodation and vocational rehabilitation.

workers and their families, unions, health care providers) suggests that the costs and consequences borne by stakeholders in their full variety ought to be considered (see Chapter 2 for a discussion of perspective). This is the norm for economic evaluations in other areas that have multiple stakeholders, such as assessments of environmental impacts. A broad perspective does not preclude providing information on specific stakeholder perspectives. In fact, a disaggregation of the costs and consequences and their re-aggregation according to stakeholder can provide invaluable insight into the distribution of burdens and benefits, and provide an indication of those who are likely to support or oppose an intervention.

Consideration of the perspective of individual stakeholders and a broad (societal) one provides insight into potential double counting traps. In some cases, the costs and consequences accruing to some stakeholders may simply be a transfer from others. For example, the wage replacement benefits saved by an insurer due to the prevention of work disability are partially or fully offset by reduced premiums billed to firms if premiums are experience rated. While it is important to distinguish between social costs and transfers, failure to identify gainers and losers, even when the gains and losses balance out in terms of dollars, is to fail to provide information that might be of significant importance to some stakeholders. The fairly conventional practice of assuming that a dollar lost to one group is exactly offset by a dollar gain to another also implies the rightness of assigning an equal weight per dollar gained or lost. The rightness or wrongness of such an assignment will be context dependent and, in general, worth exploring with decision makers to see whether differential distributional weights might be advised (see Chapter 13 on equity for details).

Figure 10.1 in Chapter 10 identifies the costs and consequences associated with an OHS intervention and the stakeholders to whom they might commonly accrue. It identifies three broad categories of stakeholders: 1) firm owners; 2) the public sector (e.g. ministries with OHS legislative, oversight and service provision responsibilities) and insurance providers (e.g., health care insurers, short-term and long-term disability insurance providers, other pension providers); and 3) workers and their families. This is not a comprehensive list but it does include those usually considered most relevant.

Workers' compensation benefits are not listed in Figure 10.1, since these are transfers from the societal perspective. At the societal level, *ex ante*, premiums are paid by employers to insurers to cover future wage replacement benefits, administration, health care, rehabilitation and other claims costs. *Ex post*, a portion is transferred from insurers to workers for the purpose of wage replacement. These transfers do not change the aggregate value of resources available to society. In general, transfers reflect a redistribution of resources, but no change in their overall availability at the societal level. However, at the individual stakeholder level they are relevant, as we have seen, and one may be interested in tracking them in order to understand their implications for stakeholders.

For an employer and the OHS system, the impact of changes in insurance obligations matter, and it is to be included in the accounting of costs and consequences. Specifically, the premium setting process for workers' compensation insurance may be experience rated to varying degrees, so a fraction of changes in the cost of occupational injuries and diseases may be realized by the firm through adjustment to its premiums. Some changes may be realized in whole or in part by all firms in the industry or rate group, and some may be realized by the insurer in the form of changes in retained earnings/profits. At the firm level it is the impact on firm premiums that matter, at the system level it is the impact on systems resources, and at the societal level it is the net change in societal burden.

On a practical level, there may be cost shifting between different types of disability insurance programmes. The burden of occupational injury and disease may be shifted to varying degrees from workers' compensation to other disability and health care programmes, unemployment insurance, and/or public pension plans depending on a variety of factors. A key factor may be the generosity of benefits to workers and the cost to employers of alternative programmes. Needless to say, it is important for researchers evaluating an intervention to look more broadly at the range of insurance and social programmes available to workers and employers, in order to identify the full extent of consequences and their distribution across stakeholders.

The consequences of occupational injury and disease

Figure 11.1 classifies work disability and other losses experienced by a worker from an occupational injury and disease. The schema distinguishes between fatalities and work disability, and between impairment and work disability. A further distinction is between work disability and disabilities associated with other social roles. Finally, the schema highlights the possible extent of losses that might follow from each category of disability. As is apparent from Figure 11.1, losses can extend beyond work productivity losses and beyond what is compensated through workers' compensation.

A more detailed description of the principal consequences of occupational injury and disease can highlight the values that might be created and resources saved through an OHS intervention.

Workers experience pain, suffering, and loss of enjoyment of life from ailments associated with occupational injury and disease. Out-of-pocket costs

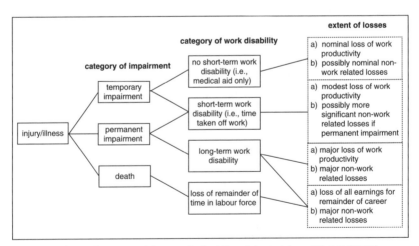

Fig. 11.1 Schema for categorizing work disability. Adapted from Weil D (2001). Valuing the economic consequences of work injury and illness: a comparision of methods and findings. *American Journal of Industrial Medicine*, 40, pp. 418–37.

may be incurred for travel to receive health care, and for products and services not covered by workers' compensation. Workers and their families will also incur time costs, which are often taken away from time used to perform non-work roles. Consequently, values created in domestic work, parenting, community, and leisure roles will be reduced. Family members may also take time off work to tend the worker, so the carers' work productivity may, in turn, also decrease. Some substitution of role performance may occur at the family level to mitigate losses. For example, in the short term, an injured worker may be able to perform some domestic chores to allow other family members more time for work roles. Longer-term losses may be substantial in cases of permanent impairment and long-term work disability. For example, someone sustaining a permanent impairment at a young age may have substantially reduced educational opportunities and so have a lifetime of lower earning power. Even short-term injuries and diseases that do not result in permanent impairment can give rise to long-term earnings losses due to factors such as loss of seniority, loss of valuable work experience and stigmatization because of the incident (Boden and Galizzi 1999).

When an occupational injury or disease occurs, the production process may be slowed down and/or halted temporarily. The worker's own time may be taken away from the production process, as might be co-workers' time. There may be other costs to the firm, such as equipment repair or replacement, particularly if the incident is associated with substantial equipment damage. If the worker is absent from work on paid leave, the production of that worker will be lost unless the effect is mitigated by hiring a replacement worker, having co-workers take up the slack or having the worker put in extra time upon return to work. These efforts may not fully recoup all losses in the short term, and replacing factors of production may carry additional costs beyond recruiting. For example, wages may have premiums attached, such as overtime pay and temporary employment agency service fees. Once back at work presenteeism may be a concern: the injured worker may not be fully recovered and, hence, there may be continued productivity losses in the short-term. Presenteeism can also precede absenteeism, that is, an occupational injury or disease may reduce productivity prior to absence. In other cases there may not be an absence at all, but simply increased presenteeism. With mental health conditions, such as stress and depression, presenteeism may be an issue without the occurrence of an absence. Additionally, if a compensation claim is made, it will require management and human resources time to administer, and may also result in possible expenses to the firm over and above increases in insurance premiums associated with occupational injury or disease. Other business values may also be affected, such as good will, reputation, and social

Box 11.2 Categories of potential losses at the firm level

Repair/replacement of damaged equipment, tools, and facilities
Loss of use of equipment while it is being repaired
Material expenses
Production delays including other workers' time
Management time dealing with the incident
Expenses associated with government investigation orders
Production delays associated with possible stop-work orders
Legal expenses if charges laid
Payment of fines

capital, particularly if the incident appears to be due to negligence on the part of the firm. Box 11.2 provides a more detailed list of possible firm-level losses (Workplace Safety and Insurance Board of Ontario and Canadian Manufacturers and Exporters 2002).

At the public sector/system level, the Ministry of Labour may experience increased programme administration and delivery costs due to greater demands on inspectorate resources. An insurer incurs costs associated with the administration of claims and the provision of health care, wage replacement and physical and vocational rehabilitation in cases of more serious injuries and diseases. Many of these costs are paid for by firms through premiums that may be, at least in part, experience rated.

At the macro-economic level, disability and related costs may ultimately affect private consumption, domestic production and national income. Disability may also have implications for labour supply and unemployment, which in turn has implications for wages, labour costs and competitiveness, and national income (Koopmanschap *et al.* 1995). Judgment will have to be exercised as to the significance of such considerations in the context of any specific study.

The above description of the consequences of occupational injury and disease may generate a long list of items for consideration. We have selected the consequences that seem most frequently to arise and the stakeholders with whom they are mainly associated: firms, the public sector and insurance providers, and workers and their families. How best to capture these consequences and what metrics to use will depend on the nature of the intervention, the context and purpose of the evaluation, the perspective taken, the projected distribution of consequences across stakeholders, and various practical considerations such as the feasibility of data collection and resources likely to be available for the evaluation. Distributive equity is likely an important practical factor in assessing the desirability of the intervention and raises its own analytical challenges if it is to be incorporated into the evaluation (see Chapter 13).

Distinguishing between health and productivity consequences

The productivity consequences of health improvements are sometimes included within the health outcome measure, or they can be measured as a distinct consequence of the intervention. One must be conscious of how these consequences are captured in order to avoid double counting, or inadvertently not including them at all. This is particularly so with cost–benefit analysis (CBA) and cost–utility analysis (CUA) since, when individuals are asked to value health states in monetary or utility terms (e.g., through contingent valuation or utility solicitation exercises), respondents' own productivity implications may have already been incorporated into those valuations unless respondents are explicitly asked to ignore them (see Gold *et al.* 1996, pp. 181–3; Drummond *et al.* 2005, pp. 78–88). In other forms of CBA, especially the human capital and revealed preference approaches, individuals' productivity implications are directly included in the valuation of health states. The human capital approach is based on the notion that the value of healthy time is determined primarily by the productivity of that time. The revealed preference approach, in principle, captures the productivity consequences in the compensating wage differentials paid to workers for assuming health risks (see Chapter 5). With cost-effectiveness analysis (CEA), productivity consequences are generally not captured in the outcome measure, though in some cases they may be, as with disability days or activities of daily living measures.

Incorporating monetary measures of productivity into economic evaluations will, all else being equal, result in larger estimates of value in programmes directed at the working population and, within working populations, at those earning higher incomes. There are often distributional issues that might not be apparent unless explicitly drawn out by the analysis and failure to address them can lead to results that (probably inadvertently) exacerbate health and income inequalities. For example, in CBA, the human capital approach expressly gives more value to high income earners since it uses market wages to value health. In the same vein, contingent valuation estimates are determined in part by ability to pay. Hence, the value of health benefits to individuals with a higher willingness to pay due to their greater ability to pay will have higher empirical estimates than those of individuals with lower incomes. The revealed prefer-ence approach for monetizing health values also results in higher estimates of the value of benefits for high income groups for the same reason. If health is measured in non-monetary terms, as in CEA and CUA, then monetized pro-ductivity changes might be measured as a separate consequence and included in the numerator of the cost-effectiveness or cost–utility ratio, with cost reducing consequences being deducted from the positive costs.

With CUA, some researchers suggest using utility elicitation to capture the value of health in all areas other than labour-market activity (e.g., for the value of reduced pain, suffering and the loss of enjoyment of life, and the value of increased time for roles other than work), and coupling this with a money metric for the productivity implications (Brouwer *et al.* 1997; Weil 2001; Drummond *et al.* 2005). Drummond *et al.* (2005) also suggest that productivity consequences be reported separately from the principal intervention costs and consequences in health care evaluations. This is to enable the implications of including productivity in an evaluation to be made explicit. The same approach should be taken in evaluations of OHS interventions, where productivity consequences are often of key interest to the firm. Knowledge of the magnitude of these consequences is therefore a poten-tially important factor in the firm's decision of whether to implement an intervention.

If the costs and consequences at the firm level imply that the intervention is not worth undertaking for the firm, but is worthwhile at the societal level, then subsidization by the public sector or regulation might be considered. However, whether it is worthwhile at the societal level depends, of course, on having knowledge of all the costs and consequences, including the productivity consequences. The same information is needed to understand the extent to which a minority perspective diverges from the societal and the amount of the subsidy (or the character of the regulation) that would be required to make implementation desirable (or effective) for the firm.

In the following sections we describe different approaches to the measure-ment of health and productivity consequences. We discuss three categories of metrics—monetary, natural, and utility-based—as used, respectively, in CBA, CEA and CUA. The generic issues related to the measurement of health and productivity consequences in CBA, CEA, and CUA are widely discussed elsewhere (e.g. Gold *et al.* 1996; Haddix *et al.* 2003; Drummond *et al.* 2005). We concentrate here on the aspects of their application most salient to OHS interventions. We also provide examples from the OHS research litera-ture on interventions in actual workplaces to illustrate the application of the theory.

Monetary measurement of consequences

There are three generic methods for quantifying the health and productivity consequences of occupational injury and disease in monetary terms: the human capital approach, the revealed preference approach, and the stated preference approach (contingent valuation).

The human capital approach for valuing consequences suggests that productive time is the primary value flowing from good health. The approach assumes full employment (usually only implicitly), and that it is impossible to replace injured or ill workers from the ranks of the unemployed. In the absence of an intervention, productivity losses are assumed to continue until return to work, or in the case of permanent work disability and death, until age of retirement, so there is a very strong zero-substitution assumption that is more or less permanent. Koopmanschap *et al.* (1995) describe the human capital approach as a measure of potential productivity losses, and it would certainly seem to generate an upper-bound estimate in the long run. In the short run, losses might actually exceed the wage cost of the absence due to the disruption in the production process resulting from the occupational injury or disease.

Essentially, the human capital approach is an estimate of the counterfactual, that is, what the individual would have earned or produced had they not been injured or ill. Actual wages are used to calculate labour-market losses and assumed to be either fixed over time (this is the basis on which many worker compensation wage replacement programmes operate) or adjusted for lifetime earnings growth. Adjustments are based on data from population statistics (stratified where desired by occupation, educational attainment, and other relevant labour-market earnings characteristics) or collected through matching of injured individuals with a healthy cohort on sociodemographic characteristics and contextual factors that bear on earnings potential (see Weil 2001 for a summary of methods). For non-wage work, the opportunity cost of time or replacement cost approach might be used to estimate potential productivity losses in non-work roles (see Drummond *et al.* 2005, p. 216 for details).

There are three key concerns regarding the human capital approach. First, wage rates may not accurately reflect the marginal product of a worker due to market imperfections. Second, its focus on productivity as the only source of health related utility is too narrow by many accounts. Third, the strong assumptions about no substitution possibilities in the production function, even in the long run, are not well founded.

The revealed preference approach uses compensating wage differentials negotiated between employers and workers to estimate wage-health risk tradeoffs (see Chapter 5; Viscusi 1993; Dorman 1996; Dorman and Hagstrom 1998). Revealed preferences are held to generally encapsulate all the knowable consequences arising from on-the-job health risks (i.e., both health and productivity), as well as other undesirable aspects of a job that are unrelated to health, such as the griminess of a job. This approach is not often used in economic evaluations for several reasons: the values found in different studies have proved to be mutually inconsistent; it is difficult to disentangle the interrelated factors bearing on the wage differentials; and factors that might distort the differentials are usually present, such as labour-market imperfections.

The contingent valuation or stated preference approach (willingness-to-pay and willingness-to-accept) uses survey methods to collect data on respondents' preferences, specifically their maximum willingness to pay for different programmes or outcomes, or their willingness to accept money in lieu of desirable programmes or outcomes. It can be used to value all consequences or simply the health component alone (e.g., health outcomes, treatments, earlier access to treatment programmes). A more restricted willingness-to-pay approach that exclusively values health consequences would be consistent with our later recommendations for a utility-elicitation approach. We are unaware of any OHS intervention evaluations that have used the contingent valuation approach. In contrast, there has been a rapid growth in the number of such studies in health technology assessment (HTA).

Monetary measurement focused exclusively on productivity consequences

If productivity consequences are measured separately, they are either embodied in the net present value in a CBA, or included in the numerator of a cost-effectiveness or cost–utility ratio as either additional costs or offsets to other costs. This is a mere convention; productivity effects, whether positive or negative, are consequences. In general, locating elements in either the numerator or the denominator of a ratio will affect the value of the ratio and, therefore, explicitness is essential to ensure misleading comparisons are not made with other studies or with a threshold ratio. In all cases, it is recommended to report the productivity consequences separately, as well as including them in the analysis, in order to make explicit their magnitude and impact on the net monetary amounts (i.e., net present value or net cost in the numerator of a ratio). Box 11.3 provides a formulation of CBA, CEA, and CUA with productivity identified as a separate measure (see Drummond *et al.* 2005, pp. 17–25 for a detailed exposition). In this section we focus on the conceptual issues and measurement options for the component labelled 'net productivity gains' in Box 11.3.

Box 11.3 Formulation of summary measures in CBA, CEA, and CUA with separate measurement of productivity

CBA: net present value = monetary value of health state changes + net productivity gains—costs of the intervention

CEA: cost-effectiveness ratio = (costs of the intervention—net productivity gains)/health effects in natural units

CUA: cost–utility ratio = (costs of the intervention—net productivity gains)/health preferences in QALYs

Historically, the human capital approach was used to measure productivity consequences of health improvements, although more recent work has concentrated on methods reflecting consequences at the firm and societal levels, as well as the short- and long-term implications for aggregate productivity. Many evaluation studies in the OHS literature taking the perspective of the firm still use the human capital approach. These studies are usually concerned only with the measurement of the productivity consequences of the intervention and do not consider the value of health to workers separately (i.e., they undertake a CBA using the human capital approach without including a monetary value of health state changes as a distinct measure).

In considering how a work absence might affect a firm's productivity, we describe the key factors that might bear on the magnitude of these consequences. A firm's adjustment to an occupational injury or disease can be achieved in various ways, depending on the nature of production process and the duration of absence (short-term vs. long-term). With short-term absences, some work can be postponed, some might be taken over by colleagues (during regular work hours or on an overtime basis) and some might be completed by a replacement worker from internal labour reserves or from a temporary employment agency. With longer-term absences, a temporary or permanent replacement may be hired or the extra work can be distributed among the existing staff by cutting less time-sensitive work.

If the firm maintains its production rates during the early period of the absence, it may, as we have seen, incur additional costs such as overtime payment for other employees, a premium for temporary replacement workers, or the costs of hiring a permanent replacement worker and associated incremental costs such as training costs. The total value of these productivity related consequences during this period will consist of the value of lost production (if any), the additional labour costs and recruiting and training costs. The length of the early period of losses will depend on the state and efficiency of the labour market, as well as the occupation of the injured worker, the industry in question, and the associated learning time required for a new recruit to get up to speed. If the level of unemployment in the economy as a whole is higher than the level of frictional unemployment, firms will be able to replace injured workers more readily. Identifying whether the unemployment rate exceeds the frictional level may be a challenge, although on average unemployment has been sufficiently high in most developed economies over the last two decades for it to have probably exceeded the frictional rate for much of the time. Additionally, firms have increasingly relied on flexible hiring practices, such as temporary and on-call contracts and temporary employment agency hires, thus providing them with a pool of backup labour to adjust to market shocks (see Tompa *et al.* 2007a for review of the literature).

The 'friction cost approach' (Koopmanschap *et al.* 1995) is one approach to measuring the productivity consequences of health improvements at the aggregate level. According to this approach there is a short-run friction period during which a firm and society may incur losses as an adjustment is made to a worker's absence. In the long run no losses are held to occur because the injured worker either returns to work and performance returns to the pre-injury level, or the firm replaces the injured worker with a new hire and performance eventually becomes comparable to what it was before. Box 11.4

Box 11.4 Friction cost and human capital approaches

Koopmanschap *et al.* (1995, Table 2, p. 182) used data from the Netherlands and compared the friction cost and human capital approaches to demonstrate the divergence in values derived under each approach. A comparison is made of the indirect cost of disease in the Netherlands in 1988 in billions of Dutch guilders.

Cost category	Friction cost approach	Human capital approach
Absence from work	9.2	23.8
Disability	0.15	49.1
Mortality	0.15	8.0

As is apparent, the friction cost approach consistently identifies much smaller productivity losses than the human capital approach.

provides an overview of the analysis using both the friction cost and human capital approaches applied to data from the Netherlands.

A group of researchers in the United States have also undertaken conceptual and empirical work on the productivity consequences of absences (Pauly *et al.* 2002). They postulate that the productivity losses of absence are generally greater than the wage rate. This is in contrast to the conceptual work and empirical results presented above. Pauly and colleagues identified three principal characteristics that determine the size and distribution of productivity losses due to work absence: the extent to which the production process relies on team work, the size of penalty incurred for not achieving target output levels, and the costs of replacing an absent worker with an equally productive worker.

Under full employment, the wage rate is a good measure of productivity losses where there is a perfect substitute for a worker at the same wage rate. The value of productivity losses due to absence exceeds the wage rate if a replacement worker is less productive or costs more than the wage rate, and the production process relies on team work or there is a penalty incurred for failing to achieve output targets. Under less than full employment, the prevailing wage rate may differ from the equilibrium wage rate, so the firm, worker, and societal values of labour time may differ. If this difference is small, the productivity losses from absence would be similar to the full employment case. An application of this framework based on data from the US can be found in Nicholson *et al.* (2006). They estimated that the median wage multiplier (defined as the day cost to a firm of an absence as a proportion of the daily wage) was 1.28, supporting the proposition by Pauly and colleagues that true absence costs are generally greater than the wage rate and, of course, further widening the gap between the friction cost and the human capital methods.

More recent work on the productivity costs of health have focussed on including consideration of losses from presenteeism (Brouwer *et al.* 2002). A variation of the friction cost approach recognizes that a period of reduced performance might occur before or after a health-related work absence, or both, or that there might simply be a period of reduced performance without an absence due to poor health. Brouwer *et al.* (2002) examined data from a Dutch trade firm and found that productivity losses due to reduced performance at work accounted for about 14% of total productivity losses.

The literature on measuring health-related at-work performance (presenteeism) is still relatively young, though its volume is growing rapidly. Examples of studies that consider productivity losses due to reduced at-work performance include Osterhaus *et al.* (1992), Burton *et al.* (1999), Berndt *et al.* (2000), and DeRango *et al.* (2003). Box 11.5 provides an example from one of these studies.

Box 11.5 A study of productivity due to absence and reduced at-work performance

A study by Burton *et al.* (1999) examined the association between health risk factors and worker productivity using administrative data from a call centre. A Worker Productivity Index was derived to capture both lost productivity due to absence and reduced at-work performance to represent the total amount of time per full-time work week that an employee was effectively productive.

The study found that productivity losses due to presenteeism (3.8 hours lost per week on average) were far greater than those due to absenteeism (0.5 hours lost per week on average). It also found that the greater the number of health risk factors, the lower the productivity of the worker.

Consequences in natural units

Some studies have focused on a range of intermediate and final outcome measures in natural units, such as safety behaviour, training, pain, discomfort, symptoms, general health status, cases of particular health conditions, injuries, diseases, and number and severity of injuries and diseases. Table 11.1 provides a glimpse of the range of measures used in the literature, drawn from a systematic review of participatory ergonomics interventions (Rivilis *et al.* 2008).

Measures can be classified as specific or general, that is, specific to a particular health condition or a measure of general health. They may also be categorized as intermediate or final, that is, intermediate proxies for downstream health outcomes or direct measures of end-state and ultimate outcomes. Choice of measure(s) depends on the purpose and context of the study. Ideally, the objective of the intervention should indicate the types of measure that are worth considering. In some cases more than one will be appropriate, as when there are multiple objectives or when a range of measures together provides a more complete assessment of the health consequences of interest than a single measure. Intermediate measures may also be useful to include along with final outcome measures when the study's measurement time frame is relatively short and it is uncertain whether a discernable impact on final outcomes will be obtainable. The availability of data from administrative sources and the resources available for primary data collection may restrict the range of options. The usual experience is that data availability is very limited in many firms, that the feasibility of extensive primary data collection is also

Table 11.1 Health outcome measures and other characteristics of studies included in a systematic review of participatory ergonomics interventions (Rivilis *et al.* 2008).

Author(s)	Jurisdiction	Industry/sector	Study design	Health outcome measures
Carrivick *et al.* (2001)	Victoria, Australia	Health care	Before–after with three comparison groups	Lost-time injury Lost-time injury duration
Evanoff *et al.* (1999)	Missouri, United States	Health care	Before–during–after	Symptoms related to discomfort Injuries
Halpern and Dawson (1997)	Colorado, United States	Automotive—accessories plant	Before–after	Injuries
Ketola *et al.* (2002)	Espoo, Finland	Government—municipal office	Individual randomized trial	MSK discomfort Pain/strain in the last 30 days
Laitinen *et al.* (1997)	Finland	Transportation—state railway metal working shop	Before–after	Sick leave
Lanoie and Tavenas (1996)	Quebec, Canada	Food—alcohol distributor	Before–during–after	Lost-time back injuries
Moore and Garg (1997)	Mid-west, United States	Food—red meat packer	Before–after	MSK injuries Lost-time injuries
Morken *et al.* (2002)	Norway	Primary—aluminium manufacturer	Group randomized trial	MSK injuries
Reynolds *et al.* (1994)	Pennsylvania, United States	Textiles—apparel manufacturer	Before–after	Body part discomfort by area Lost-time injuries
Wickström *et al.* (1993)	Finland	Primary—metal manufacturer	Before–after	Low back pain in past 12 months Sick leave due to low-back pain

low, and that the length of time required between exposures and effects on final health outcomes is too long to be observed in practice. Intermediate measures are the practical, although imperfect, response to these limitations. In all such cases, given an absence of available modelling skills and the data to which to apply them, professional and managerial judgment will usually be needed to make a link between the intermediate outcomes and final outcomes. Formal methods, such as Delphi techniques or consensus conferences might be used to elucidate these links.

The intermediate and final outcome measures commonly used in OHS interventions, such as pain, symptoms, cases of particular injuries and diseases, lost-time and no-lost-time claim counts, and disability days averted, may be convenient to use in an economic evaluation if they are easily attainable, but the lack of comparability (generalizability) is a concern. Even when studies use similar outcomes, they may not be fully comparable because different measurement protocols have been used, such as pain being measured using different questionnaires with different scales. General health measures such as SF-36 are more broadly applicable and comparable, and have been tested for construct validity and reliability. However, such generic measures may be less responsive to the interventions than purpose-specific measures, particularly in the short run. In cases where there is trade-off between sensitivity of a measure to the effects of the intervention and generalizability, the need for sensitivity should take precedence, since all may be for naught if the intervention's effect on health is not drawn out.

A CEA will provide information on the incremental costs for a unit of incremental effect of a particular intervention relative to some alternative. If both the numerator (the incremental costs) and the denominator (the incremental effects) are positive, an analyst will need to determine whether the extra effect is worth the extra cost (i.e., whether the intervention is cost-effective). To assist with this assessment the analyst might turn to explicit information on a decision maker's or society's willingness to pay or some decision rule based on policy, past decisions, the costs of similar outcomes from other initiatives, or other external marker that provides guidance on the monetary value placed on a unit of effect (see Chapter 9 for detailed discussion on decision rule).

One might consider converting intermediate measures into final outcome measures, natural units into utility units, or natural units into monetary units whenever there is an acceptable understanding of the link between them. It is not good practice implicitly to assume that there is a constant and equal relationship between different types of outcome measures, that is, that a 1% change in one will lead to a 1% change in the other. Converting intermediate measures into final outcome measures may be warranted in studies where the measurement time frame is too short to observe and measure changes in final outcomes. In such cases, the analyst might use intermediate measures and convert these into final outcomes in the analysis (see Box 11.6 for an example). It is critical that the underlying assumptions made in undertaking the conversion be supported with evidence. Too often, conversion is made without explicitly stating the assumptions or without supporting the assumptions with evidence (Tompa *et al.* 2006).

The conversion from natural units into a utility-based measure is another option to consider. Drummond *et al.* (2005, p. 126) review it, although

Box 11.6 A study using intermediate outcome measures

Rempel *et al.* (2006) evaluated two workstation interventions for upper body pain and musculoskeletal disorders among computer operators. Key outcomes were pain severity and incidence of musculoskeletal disorders of the arm and neck.

Reduction in incidence of arm/shoulder cases identified
in the intervention: 49%

Workers' compensation claim rate for neck/shoulder
cases prior to the study: 0.0144

Average claim cost prior to the study: $11,540 US

Proportionate decreases of incidence identified in the study were translated into reduced workers' compensation claims for neck and shoulder disorders assuming an equally proportionate decrease. Based on this assumption the payback period for the intervention was estimated to be 10.6 months.

ultimately they caution that more research is required to refine the methods by which to do so.

The conversion from natural units into monetary units using shadow prices is regularly undertaken in OHS intervention research (see Boxes 11.6 and 11.7 for examples). For example, disability days averted may be changed to monetary units based on the wage rate of the workers affected by the intervention. As with the conversion from intermediate into final outcomes, here, too, evidence is required to support the values used in the conversion. The monetary value of specific outcomes can be taken from the firm's own data sources or from external sources that are comparable (e.g., other studies evaluating the same intervention that have used monetary measures, studies of the willingness to pay for the outcome of interest, data from national statistical agencies). In some cases it may be useful to undertake a CEA in parallel with a CBA, since the natural units may be more meaningful to users of the research than the monetary values assigned to them (and the results may be more generalizable). Including a CEA allows a reader to assess the cost-effectiveness with other monetary values for outcome measure that are more relevant to setting for which the intervention is being considered. Box 11.7 provides an example of a study that undertakes both a CEA and a CBA.

Since intermediate and final health outcome measures generally do not incorporate productivity consequences or other values created and resources saved, these are best measured separately in monetary terms and included in the numerator of the cost-effectiveness ratio. That is the approach taken in the

Box 11.7 A study with CEA and CBA

Loisel *et al.* (2002) undertook a CEA and a CBA of a treatment program for sub-acute occupational back pain from the perspective of the workers' compensation board in Quebec, Canada. The study had four arms: standard care, occupational rehabilitation treatment; clinical treatment, and a combined clinical–occupational treatment arm known as the 'Sherbrooke model'.

The key outcome in the study was the number of disability days on compensation due to back pain. Program delivery costs and consequence of disease costs were the key costs considered in the analysis. The latter refers to the costs associated with wage replacement. A standard wage replacement rate was used, which was based on the average income of workers in the control arm. Total consequence of disease costs were calculated as the number of disability days on compensation times the standard wage replacement rate.

Consequence of disease costs were included in the numerator of the CEA and in the net present value (NPV) calculations of the CBA. Incremental cost-effectiveness ratios and NPVs were calculated for the three experimental arms compared to the standard care arm at one year and 6.4 years follow-up.

study described in Box 11.7. It is also recommended that the productivity consequences be reported separately in order to make their magnitudes explicit.

It is critical to include the productivity consequences in an evaluation, since failing to do so will present a biased picture of the consequences of an intervention. Furthermore, these consequences can be an important motivator in a firm's decision to undertake an OHS intervention, so not including them in an analysis would overlook a critical factor that bears on the merits of alternative options as perceived by those who are responsible for implementing them.

Utility-based measures of consequences

We use the term 'utility-based' to refer to health-related quality of life measures that combine the quality and quantity of health. These include Quality-Adjusted Life-Years (QALYs) and variants such as Healthy Year Equivalents (HYEs), Disability-Adjusted Life-Years (DALYs), and preference-based multi-attribute health status classifications systems, such as Quality of Well-Being, and Health Utility Index.

To date, QALYs are not a measure used in the OHS literature. In a systematic review (Tompa *et al.* 2007b) we were unable to find any examples of its application in an economic evaluation of an OHS intervention. In contrast, QALYs are used extensively in the health care field. Much has been written about the basics and details of such measures for health care programme evaluation, so we focus on issues most salient to OHS interventions, namely those related to the measurement and inclusion of changes in worker time available for productive activities and the impact of interventions on aggregate (firm/societal level) productivity (see Gold *et al.* 1996 and Drummond *et al.* 2005, for a detailed presentation of the use of utility-based measures and specifically QALYs in health care intervention evaluation).

There have been ongoing discussions in the literature about how and where to capture worker time costs and aggregate productivity consequences associated with health improvements in CUA (see Gold *et al.* 1996, pp. 38–45; Brouwer *et al.* 1997, 2002; Drummond *et al.* 2005, p. 86). By 'how' we are referring to what measures to use and details of the measurement process, and by 'where' we are referring to whether to include them in the numerator (the cost measure) or denominator (the consequence measure) of a cost–utility ratio. Key concerns are to avoid double counting and to ensure all time costs and productivity consequences are accounted for in the analysis.

A list of some of the principal time costs and productivity consequences warranting consideration in the evaluation of an intervention that improves health includes:

1) changes in worker time available to generate labour-market income due to reduced morbidity and extension of life;

2) changes in worker time available for use in other social roles;

3) changes in worker time used for seeking health care treatment;

4) changes in time use by worker's family members (e.g., reduced care giving role);

5) changes in productivity at the firm and societal level;

6) changes in employer insurance premiums due to reduced injuries, diseases and fatalities;

7) changes in transfer payments provided as wage replacement;

8) changes in health care, rehabilitation and other services provided by an insurer;

9) changes in future health care and other costs in the added years of life.

The first three categories of changes are best captured in the utility elicitation process. Specifically, respondents should be asked to consider, in addition to pain, suffering, and loss of enjoyment of life, the following: the income replacement they would be entitled to, given the nature and cause of the health condition (i.e., workers' compensation, private disability insurance benefits, public disability insurance benefits, etc.); their time/productivity losses in social roles other than work; and the time lost to receiving health care. This is consistent with suggestions of several researchers (Weil 2001; Weinstein *et al.* 1997).

The fourth category, changes in time use by family members, is generally not included in the health-state preference elicitation process since the focus is on an individual's preferences for her/himself. Gold and colleagues suggest including family members' time used to provide care in the numerator, valued at the opportunity cost of their time (proxied by the wage rate). In principle, other time reallocations of family members (e.g., reallocation of time between work and non-work roles) should also be included in the numerator.

The fifth category is the productivity consequences associated with firm/societal level changes in injuries, diseases, and fatalities. These consequences should be measured using the friction cost approach and counted in the numerator. We also recommend reporting the value of firm/societal level productivity changes separately in order to make their magnitude explicit.

The sixth to eighth categories are associated with the changes in reserves required by the insurer to cover transfers to workers for wage-replacement benefits, and health care, rehabilitation, and other service costs. These are real changes in required systems- or societal-level resources to cover insurance obligations, and are reflected to varying degrees as changes in premiums to employers and changes in retained earnings/profits of insurers. Ultimately, they are changes in resources available to society and should be counted in the numerator.

The ninth category, changes in future health care and other costs incurred by the worker due to an increased length of life, present a whole new set of resource implications that could be taken into consideration [for a detailed discussion on this topic, see Gold *et al.* (1996, pp. 45–48)]. In principle, these costs should be included in the numerator, but in practice are difficult to quantify.

We have addressed all of the nine items listed above to varying degrees. To reiterate for clarity, our recommendations are as follows:

1) worker time available to generate labour-market income due to reduced morbidity or averted mortality: elicit preference scores for health states

based on assumption that wage-replacement rates will be received, where applicable;

2) worker time available for use in other social roles due to reduced morbidity: elicit preference scores for health states with respondent considering the consequence for time available for other social roles;

3) worker time used for seeking medical treatment: elicit preference scores for health states with respondent considering these time costs;

4) time use by workers' family members: quantify separately if possible, and include in the numerator;

5) firm- or societal-level responses to absence of injured worker: measure friction costs at the firm or societal level and report separately; include in the numerator;

6) insurance premiums paid by employers due to changes in injury and disease rates: include premium changes in the numerator;

7) payments provided as wage replacement: only include portion not reflected in premium changes to firms;

8) health care, rehabilitation and other services provided by an insurer: only include portion not reflected in premium changes to firms;

9) future health care and other costs in the added years of life: quantify separately if possible, and include in the numerator.

Recommendations

Following are our recommendations for good practice for the valuing of consequences:

+ Be alert to the possibility that occupational injury and disease costs may be shifted from one programme/stakeholder to another.

+ Be explicit about the range of costs that arise from occupational injury and disease and that represent possible benefits if averted.

+ Measure, when possible, the value of health separately from averted productivity costs.

+ Consider the friction cost approach if measuring averted productivity costs separately from health.

+ Be alert to the risk of double counting productivity consequences in measures of health effects, or inadvertently not including them at all.

+ Be explicit, when valuing health and productivity consequences in monetary terms, about the method used to value them (human capital, revealed-preference, or stated-preference) and use it consistently, bearing in mind the very significant differences in results that each can give.

- Be alert to the risk of biasing measures of gain or loss by use of techniques that reflect ability to pay.

- Be alert to the possibility of productivity losses through presenteeism as well as absenteeism.

- Consider including consequences of the intervention occurring beyond the measurement time frame and be explicit about how they are formulated.

- Present disaggregated consequences by category for each stakeholder separately in addition to the summary measure.

- Adjust monetary consequences for inflation so that all estimates are in constant prices (see Chapter 12 for details).

- Discount monetary and non-monetary consequences using an appropriate discount rate (see Chapter 12 for details).

- Test the impact of various assumptions about consequences through sensitivity analysis (see Chapter 12 for details).

- Undertake conversion of specific outcome measures to general ones, or intermediate to final, on the basis of the best empirical knowledge available about the relationship between them (either causal or simply an association), and never leave details of the conversion implicit or undiscussed.

- Consider using utility measures of health changes associated with OHS interventions rather than conventional morbidity or mortality data, or conventional workplace participation data.

Chapter 12

Adjusting for time preference and addressing uncertainty

William Gnam, Michel Grignon, and Roman Dolinschi

Introduction

This chapter covers two topics: adjustment for inflation and time preference, and uncertainty and sensitivity analysis. The two topics are sometimes perceived as related because the discount rate used to adjust for time preference is a parameter commonly subjected to uncertainty and, hence, subjected to sensitivity analysis. However, the issues of time preference and uncertainty are actually distinct. Hence, each is given separate treatment here. We begin the chapter with a discussion of adjustment for inflation and time preference, and follow with uncertainty and sensitivity analysis.

Part 1: adjustment for inflation and time preference

Conventional practice

Over time, nominal monetary values are typically affected by inflation. Values drawn from different years are therefore generally not directly comparable. Since the costs and monetary benefits of an intervention accrue over time, it is standard practice in economics to remove the inflationary component before comparing them. This is done by adjusting prices from different years to a base year using a price index. Price indices are available from national statistical agencies. There are often separate indices available for different categories of goods and services because they can have different rates of inflation (e.g., medical care technologies and drugs tend to increase in price from year to year at higher rates than general consumer goods and services). Hence, it is important to use indices appropriate for the goods and services under consideration.

Individuals and firms prefer to shift costs into the future, and to receive benefits early for several reasons, including a preference for consuming goods and services sooner, rather than later, uncertainty about the future, and the ability to earn interest on money received today. In general, money and resources in the future are worth less than the same quantity today. The phenomenon of preference for the timing of cost and benefits is known as 'time preference.' Because of time preference, the differential timing of resource flows across alternatives can be meaningfully compared only after translating them to a common point in time, usually the present time or the start time of the intervention. This translation of resource values to a particular point in time for the purposes of comparison is known as discounting (see Box 12.1 for an example). Adjusting resource flows for time preference is particularly relevant if the trajectory of costs and consequences over the assessment period differs between the alternatives under consideration (for detailed treatment of discounting of costs and monetary values, see Drummond *et al.* 2005, pp. 72–78 and Gold *et al.* 1996, pp. 214–219).

Note that adjustment for inflation is done for reasons different from those for adjusting for time preference, although in some cases the rate used to discount flows may include both time preference and inflation in one value. When an interest rate incorporates both time preference and inflation, the rate is often called a 'nominal interest rate', whereas a rate that does not include inflation is called the 'real interest rate.' It is preferable to address the issues of inflation and discounting separately if possible, in order to allow for the use of different rates of time preference for the purpose of sensitivity analysis, and different price indices for different categories of goods and services. Adjustment for inflation and discounting is generally not necessary if costs and benefits under consideration are incurred during a period of one year or less.

Gold *et al.* (1996) made the following recommendations about discounting:

- a standard discount rate should be used across evaluations, one that reflects a societal or planner's perspective, rather than a local or individual one;
- costs and consequences should be discounted at the same rate;
- if a jurisdiction uses an official discount rate for the valuation of public investment, this rate should be used as the standard rate for all future public investment evaluations in order to insure comparability.

Regarding the first point, the most appropriate rate will clearly depend on the perspective of the study; it is not necessarily the same for every decision maker. Regarding the second point, not all analysts agree with this recommendation; some have proposed discounting benefits at a different rate than costs. Regardless of the rate used, benefits should always be discounted even if they

Box 12.1 Adjustment for inflation and time preference example

Consider two OHS interventions (A and B) designed to reduce the incidence of repetitive strain injury in a department employing data entry clerks. Both interventions cost $40,000 over 3 years, but the cost flows differ between the two. For intervention A they are $5,000 in year 1, $5,000 in year 2, and $30,000 in year 3. For intervention B they are $30,000 in year 1, $5,000 in year 2, and $5,000 in year 3. Assume expenses occur at the end of the year and the relevant interest rate is 3%.

The generic formula for the present value of costs (PVC), adjusting cost flows from different years for both inflation and time preference is:

$$PVC = \sum_{i=1}^{n} \text{nominal cost (\$)}_{\text{year } i} / [\text{price index}_{\text{year } i} \times (1 + \text{real interest rate}_{\text{year } i})^i]$$

In our example:

Price index $_{\text{year } 1} = 1.00$, Price index $_{\text{year } 2} = 1.03$, Price index $_{\text{year } 3} = 1.05$

Real interest rate = 0.03

$PVC_A = \$5,000/[1.00 \times (1 + 0.03)] + \$5,000/[1.03 \times (1 + 0.03)^2]$
$+ \$30,000/[1.05 \times (1 + 0.03)^3] = \$35,576.98$

$PVC_B = \$30,000/[1.00 \times (1 + 0.03)] + \$5,000/[1.03 \times (1 + 0.03)^2]$
$+ \$5,000/[1.05 \times (1 + 0.03)^3] = \$38,059.74$

Since a larger fraction of the total cost is incurred earlier with intervention B relative to intervention A, its inflation adjusted and discounted total cost is higher. If the costs had simply been added together without adjustment for inflation and time preference, the two alternatives would have appeared to have been equally costly.

are measured in natural units (as in CEA) or utility adjusted units (as in CUA), otherwise postponing an intervention into the future would appear to be a better decision than undertaking it in a given time period (see Box 12.2 for a simple example, and Drummond *et al.* 2005, pp. 109–111, 189–190; Gold *et al.* 1996, pp. 214–216, 219–235 for more detailed discussions). With regard to the first and third points, a firm may have a specific discount rate pertinent to projects it considers and this may differ from the public investment rate.

Box 12.2 Discounting non-monetary benefits

If a disability management intervention has an incremental cost of $150,000 relative to the status quo, and averts 1,000 additional disability days over a period of one year, the cost-effectiveness ratio would be:

$150,000/1,000 days = $150 per disability day averted.

If it was decided to postpone the introduction of such an intervention for five years, and only costs were discounted to the present time, the intervention would appear to be less expensive per disability day averted. Assuming no inflation and a 3% discount rate, the cost-effectiveness ratio would be:

$[\$150,000/(1.03)^5]/1,000$ days = $129 per disability day averted.

Postponing the intervention even further into the future would make it appear to be even less expensive per disability day averted. However, if both costs and consequences are discounted, the cost-effectiveness ratio would not change, regardless of the planned date for introduction. In the case of a five-year delay, the cost-effectiveness ratio, with both costs and consequences discounted, is:

$[\$150,000/(1.03)^5]/[1,000$ days$/(1.03)^5] = \$150$ per disability day averted.

If this is the case both the firm specific rate and the public rate should be used in the analysis. Using a public rate will facilitate comparability with other evaluations. Gold *et al.* (1996) recommend using a discount rate of 3% per year, but since a large number of studies in the past had used a rate of 5%, they also recommend using both values for comparative purposes.

Since the publication of the Gold *et al.* (1996), a debate about the standard value for time discounting, and the practice of using the same value for both costs and consequences has been re-opened. In what follows, we present the principal aspects of this debate.

Controversy over using the same discount rate for costs and health outcomes

The debate about whether to use the same discount rate for costs and health outcomes is not specific to OHS interventions, and is still openly discussed in health technology assessment (HTA) and other economic evaluation literatures. The key issue is that the appropriate discount rate for health measured in non-monetary units may be different from that used for monetary values for several reasons. With CBA, since monetary values of health outcomes are assumed to be known at each point in time, these monetary values should be subject to the same discount rate used for costs for consistency. In contrast, with CEA and CUA we do not know the monetary equivalent of health outcomes at each point in time; therefore, quantitative health outcomes are discounted instead. If the monetary value of a unit of health is assumed to remain constant over time (for the same individual), then it would be appropriate to use the same discount rate for health outcomes as for costs, similar to CBA. However, a unit of health outcome may translate into a different monetary value depending on the point in time that the unit is received. There are many reasons why the monetary value of health might change over time, which would, in turn, have implications for the discount rate to use for quantitative health outcomes. Gravelle and Smith (2001) suggest: the rate of change for the monetary value of a unit of health outcome might stem from changes in prices of health care; the impact of prices, income and technological progress on the consumption of health care, and therefore, on the productivity of health care in the production of health; and the impact of technological progress on the productivity of health care.

It can be shown under broad assumptions that this rate of change is positive suggesting that the discount rate used for quantitative health outcomes should be smaller than the discount rate for monetary values. It can also be shown that such a rate of change will depend on the age distribution of the population to whom the programme is targeted, as well as on the initial health status of this population. Different discount rates might, therefore, very well apply to the same programme across different populations, without any assumption that the rate of time preference varies (i.e., no difference in tastes across populations is required to generate different discount rates for quantitative health outcomes).

It therefore appears that, even though CEA and CUA do not require an explicit monetary value for health outcomes, they still require some insight into the change in this value over time. Similarly, even though determining a discount rate for CBA seems straightforward in that a unique value appears to be sufficient for both costs and outcomes, there still remains the difficulty of calculating monetary values for the health outcomes at different points in time. Since we rarely know the monetary value of health outcomes at different points in time even with a CBA, it appears that the three types of economic evaluations (CBA, CEA, and CUA) face the same issue of constructing a sensible evolution of such a value over time.

If it is not practical to identify a monetary value of health outcomes at different points in time, they can be measured at the initial time period and a health outcome specific discount rate can be used. In such cases there would be two different discount rates, one for costs and one for outcomes. To determine the health outcome specific rate, an analyst might administer a questionnaire to solicit preferences from a representative population to identify the rate of exchange between future and present health outcomes (assuming, of course, that the perspective to be taken on the appropriate rate is based on the preferences of the population in question).

Part 2: uncertainty and sensitivity analysis
Sources of uncertainty in OHS interventions

OHS interventions are varied and include interventions targeted at the individual, work group, firm and system level. It is preferable to address the issues of inflation and discounting separately if possible, in order to allow for the use of different rates of time preference for the purpose of sensitivity analysis. For interventions targeted at the individual (e.g., an intervention designed to encourage early and safe return to work after an injury or illness absence), the sources and magnitude of uncertainty are likely to be similar to those of health care interventions. However, OHS interventions that occur at a higher level are similar to environmental interventions and will generally be characterized by additional sources of uncertainty. To identify sources of uncertainty that are prominent in the evaluation of OHS interventions, we draw on the taxonomies that have been described variously by Briggs (2000), Spiegelhalter *et al.* (2004), and others (see Table 12.1 for a summary of sources of uncertainty and their relative importance for OHS).

Within-individual variability

This variability arises from the unavoidable within-individual predictive uncertainty concerning specific outcomes, which manifests itself empirically as variability in outcomes between homogeneous individuals. Since the usual focus of analysis is on expected outcomes in homogeneous populations, this variability is not likely to differ between the subjects of HTA studies and those of OHS intervention studies.

Between-individual variability

With expected outcomes, this variability is generally due to the effects of identifiable subgroups of individuals who differ by age, sex, job, firm characteristics, regulatory environment, and other covariates, or who differ by unmeasured or immeasurable differences (latent variables). The heterogeneity of work-related variables is high, suggesting that this source of variability may be higher for OHS intervention evaluations than for HTA studies.

Table 12.1 Summary of sources of uncertainty.

Source of uncertainty	Details	Relative importance for OHS compared to HTA
Within-individual variability	Within-individual predictive uncertainty (or variability associated with outcomes between homogenous individuals)	Variability likely to be similar to HTA.
Between-individual variability	Variability associated with identifiable or unidentifiable characteristics	Variability may be higher due to heterogeneity of work-related characteristics.
Parameter uncertainty	Within-model uncertainty regarding the correct values of parameters	Difficult to compare, but delayed health effects of some OHS interventions, data reliability issues, and complexity of OHS environment suggest higher variability.
Model and methodological uncertainty	Uncertainty regarding the correct model and uncertainty regarding methodological choices	Likely higher due to the complexity of OHS environment and use of observational study designs. Issue of missing data, confounding, and bias add to the uncertainty. Non-linear modelling of long-term effects (e.g., Markov models) have numerous functional forms. Counterfactual of what would have happened without the intervention is sometimes not known.

Parameter uncertainty

Most of the literature on the uncertainty in HTA focuses on the within-model uncertainty about the correct values for parameters. Parameter uncertainty has been sub-classified into 'parameters that could be sampled' (i.e., parameters that could be measured accurately if sufficient evidence were available), and 'assumptions', which are qualitative judgments placed in the model that can only be made precise through some legitimate process in which a methodological template may be established.

Given the diverse nature of OHS interventions, it is not possible to make generalizations about the magnitude of parameter uncertainty in the economic evaluation of OHS interventions compared to HTA. Nonetheless, there are several sources of parameter uncertainty that arise frequently in the economic modelling of OHS safety interventions, some of which are uncommon in HTA.

First, the delayed and long-term health effects of some OHS interventions imply greater uncertainty in estimates of the magnitude of outcomes, and greater uncertainty regarding the time frame in which health effects are expected to occur. Second, there is a dearth of accurate cost and consequence information due to the fragmentation of data that may arise from the distribution of costs and consequences across different stakeholders, and from workers changing jobs, or moving between employer-based health and disability insurance systems. Finally, there are complexities associated with the OHS environment due to interrelationship between regulation, the labour market, product/service markets, and aggregate GDP that might vary in the future in ways that are hard to predict.

Model and methodological uncertainty

This type of uncertainty describes the lack of knowledge concerning the appropriate qualitative structure of the model and uncertainty regarding methodological choices when conducting an evaluation. There are several sources of uncertainty in the economic modelling of OHS interventions that are less common in HTA. Because some OHS intervention studies measure the impact of changes in the work environment on health, the complexity of issues and the use of observational, rather than experimental designs create uncertainty about the correct model for estimating causal effects. This is a pervasive feature of preventive interventions (Luken 1985). It implies relying on modelling more than when estimating the effects of curative interventions. Handling missing data, and controlling for confounding and bias with non-experimental study designs involve choices of methods and functional model forms that are uncertain. Many OHS interventions (such as interventions to alter the course of chronic industrial diseases) have lagged or long-term effects. Since observation may provide only clinical endpoints, non-multilinear methods such as Markov models may be required to simulate long-term effects. These models have numerous functional forms, with uncertainty about which one the analyst should use. Finally, universal OHS interventions (ones that include the entire workforce) create methodological problems and uncertainties in modelling outcomes, since it is uncertain what would have occurred if not for the OHS intervention. Illustrating several of these methodological uncertainties in an area with a similar range of sources of uncertainty as OHS, Fahs *et al.* (1997) wrote:

> Reversing global climate change and stratospheric ozone depletion present a particular challenge for cost-effectiveness analysis, due to the uncertainties involved not only in the general impact of efforts to reverse the process, but also the health impact via illness and mortality avoided compared with what would have happened in an alternative scenario.

Methods of handling uncertainty

Recent HTA guidelines have considered the appropriate methods for characterizing the uncertainty of cost-effectiveness estimates [Gold 1996; National Institute for Clinical Excellence (NICE) 2004]. There are several reasons why uncertainty in economic evaluations should be characterized expressly and accurately. Characterizing uncertainty can provide insight into the robustness of results under alternative scenarios, reveal additional data requirements before an intervention is widely adopted, inform future research directions, and influence the timing of a reappraisal of an evaluation in anticipation of additional evidence becoming available.

When complex models are used in economic evaluation in which there is a non-linear relationship between inputs and outputs (e.g., Markov models), an accurate calculation of expected costs and effects is required, and depends upon the full expression of uncertainty surrounding parameters. Dealing with uncertainty is important in all economic evaluations and economic evaluations of OHS interventions are no different. We present several options for assessing the impact of uncertainty on the robustness of the results from an economic evaluation. (See Table 12.2.)

Sensitivity analyses

The traditional method of characterizing uncertainty in economic evaluation studies has been through deterministic sensitivity analyses, whereby critical parameters in the model are varied over a plausible range, and the cost-effectiveness/cost–utility ratios or other outcome measures are then recalculated (Briggs *et al.* 1994). Sensitivity analyses have been conducted one variable at a time, with variables in combinations, or by identifying a set of extreme circumstances (best/worst case scenario analysis) or other scenarios across parameters that yield a range of ratios. Gold *et al.* (1996) recommended that economic analysts at a minimum conduct univariate (varying one element at a time), and bivariate or multivariate (varying two or more elements simultaneously) sensitivity analyses for important parameters, and employ statistical methods or simulation when faced with substantial uncertainty regarding parameter values. These recommendations were made before the recent proliferation of research in probabilistic sensitivity analysis (PSA), and before the growth of published applications using the method.

In contrast, the recently updated NICE guidance for HTA has endorsed PSA, arguing that deterministic sensitivity analysis can manage simultaneous analysis of only two or three variables, and underestimates the combined implications of uncertainty in parameters (NICE 2004). In the realm of economic evaluation of OHS interventions, where parameter uncertainty is

Table 12.2 Prescriptions for handling uncertainty.

Method	Strengths and limitations	Where to go for more details
Deterministic sensitivity analysis (univariate and multivariate)	Addresses uncertainty with regard to the estimate of one or more parameters Simple to undertake May underestimate the combined impact of uncertainty in parameters Multivariate sensitivity analysis can become more time and computationally burdensome Difficult to interpret if parameters have complicated correlational structures	Gold *et al.* (1996) pp. 249–261 Drummond *et al.* (2005) pp. 42–43
Classic probabilistic sensitivity analysis	More fully represents uncertainty across parameters within a model than deterministic approach Computationally more demanding Assumes distribution of parameters is known	Gold *et al.* (1996) pp. 261–263 Drummond *et al.* (2005) pp. 302–303 Claxton *et al.* (2005)
Bayesian probabilistic sensitivity analysis	Represents uncertainty across parameters within a model without assuming that distributions conform to predefined shapes Can include explicit modelling of the joint sampling distributions Correlation between unknown quantities is preserved Complexity of statistical methods requires special skills Need for special software	Gold *et al.* (1996) pp. 263–264 Spiegelhalter *et al.* (2004)
Alternate model/ methods sensitivity analysis	Addresses issue of uncertainty with regard to the correct functional form of the model and the methodological assumptions Focus on parameter uncertainty conditional on that model underestimates the true level of uncertainty If weighting analyses from different structural model assumptions, may become intractable if there are many assumptions Requires special skills	Gold *et al.* (1996) pp.267–270 Drummond *et al.* (2005) pp. 303–304 Draper (1995)

likely to be significant and greater than that found in HTA, the risk of under-estimating and misrepresenting the extent of uncertainty with deterministic sensitivity analysis may be magnified. Multivariate sensitivity analyses of multiple parameters, used to explore uncertainty with a larger number of parameters, can also be limited by time and computation burden, as well as by problems with interpretation, particularly if the parameters in the sensitivity analysis have complicated correlation structures (Claxton 2005). This suggests that deterministic sensitivity analysis is limited in its ability to characterize the uncertainty inherent in economic evaluations of OHS interventions, and that PSA, discussed below, will generally be the preferred method to characterize uncertainty in such interventions.

Probabilistic sensitivity analysis (PSA)

PSA requires that all estimates of input parameters within a model be specified as full probability distributions, rather than point estimates, in order to represent the uncertainty related to their values more fully. The distributions chosen to reflect the uncertainty for individual parameters are guided by the type of parameter, the estimation process, and the form of the data. Published examples of PSA have often assumed independence between parameters, although this is not a required assumption with the approach, and several methods exist to model correlations between parameters. Once these distributions are specified, the most common approach is to propagate parameter uncertainty through the model. The imprecision of the economic evaluation results (reflecting composite parameter uncertainty) is usually represented using such methods as cost-effectiveness acceptability curves (see Chapter 9 for details). Using PSA, the contributions of specific parameters or groups of parameters to decision uncertainty can be assessed by using value-of-information methods for individual parameters or groups of parameters (Ades 2003). In practice, the method can offer helpful guidance as to where future research might be best directed to reduce the effect of the principal causes of uncertainty.

Bayesian versus classical approaches to PSA

Although several authors and advocates of PSA have adopted an explicitly Bayesian framework, PSA can be conducted using classical statistical approaches. Our purpose in comparing Classical with Bayesian approaches is not to add further to the extensive and often polemical literature favouring one approach over the other. Rather, we have adopted the purely pragmatic strategy of describing the relative practical advantages and disadvantages of the approaches as they pertain to PSA.

PSA in a classical framework has also been described as a two-stage approach (Spiegelhalter *et al.* 2004). In the first stage, probability distributions are assigned to each of the parameters of interest based upon subjective judgments (including expert panel recommendations), data analyses, or some combination of the two. Generally, the distributions chosen for parameters are assumed to be independent and parametric. Once the distributions for each parameter have been specified, the second stage is to calculate the overall distribution of the outcome measure (e.g., the incremental cost-effectiveness ratio) by Monte Carlo simulation or by using second-order Taylor series expansion (such as the delta method) to estimate the variance of the outcome or its components. Simulation through Monte Carlo methods may be achieved using standard software, such as Microsoft Excel macros, or several commercial software packages.

In a full Bayesian framework, initial prior opinions on the distribution of the parameters are revised by Bayes theorem to posterior distributions, the effects of which are propagated through the economic model in order to make predictions. This process can include the explicit modelling of the joint sampling distribution of health effects and costs (O'Hagan and Stevens 2002). The complexity of the inferences makes Markov-Chain Monte-Carlo (MCMC) analysis the computational procedure of choice for calculating the posterior distribution. MCMC simulation methods require specialized software, such as WinBUGS.

For modelling OHS interventions, a full Bayesian approach confers several advantages. Perhaps the most important is that the appropriate correlations between unknown quantities are preserved and propagated, rather than assuming either independence, or making arbitrary assumptions such as multivariate normality. This may be particularly important in models that use highly correlated data, such as repeated observations (e.g., both baseline levels and treatment differences) from the same study. Another advantage of the full Bayesian approach is that there is no need to assume that probability distributions conform to predefined parametric shapes. In OHS interventions this may be important for inferences that involve small samples.

The primary disadvantage of the Bayesian framework is the additional complexity in the implementation and simulation of the statistical model, and the need to use MCMC software. We strongly recommend that research teams using the Bayesian economic evaluation model recruit the expertise of a statistician or econometrician experienced in MCMC simulation methods.

Alternate model/method sensitivity analyses

Uncertainty regarding the correct qualitative form of the economic evaluation model is not a unique problem to OHS interventions. Nonetheless, as noted above, the modelling of OHS interventions at higher levels such as the work group or firm level is likely to bring additional sources of uncertainty related to modelling lagged outcomes, controlling for confounding, and modelling causal effects with non-experimental study designs. The NICE guidelines recommend that these forms of uncertainty be dealt with by deterministic sensitivity analysis, whereby a separate (probabilistic) model result is created for each alternative model or major methodological assumption. Draper (1995) has argued that focusing only on parameter uncertainty conditional on a given model underestimates the true level of uncertainty. He makes the Bayesian argument that model structure itself may be subject to repeated analyses utilizing different models and specifying prior probabilities of different models across this model space. This suggestion is related to the proposed solution by Gold *et al.* (1996) who recommended appropriately weighting analyses employing different structural model assumptions. However, it is doubtful whether this recommendation is tractable for the multitude of assumptions and judgments that must be made for every economic evaluation (Briggs 2000), and it is even more doubtful that this process could be conducted by the same analysts. The costs and practical barriers in commissioning multiple teams of analysts to create the same cost-effectiveness models suggest that this recommendation is generally not feasible, particularly in light of the additional modelling uncertainty related to economic evaluation of some OHS interventions. Indeed, keeping the (deterministic) sensitivity analyses of modelling and methodological assumptions manageable requires critical judgment regarding the most important features of functional form and methodology. These considerations suggest that deterministic sensitivity analysis of modelling and methodological uncertainty remains the method of choice for economic evaluations of OHS interventions.

Recommendations

Part 1 recommendations: adjusting for inflation and time preference

- The differential timing of resource flows for alternative interventions can only be meaningfully compared by translating them to a common point in time, usually the present or the start date of the intervention.
- Adjust costs and monetary consequences occurring over multiple years for inflation.
- As a separate exercise, discount costs and monetary consequences occurring over multiple years to the start of the intervention or the time of decision to intervene.
- Discount non-monetary consequences occurring over multiple years to the start of the intervention or the time of decision to intervene.

- Use a discount rate that is relevant to the decision maker.
- Consider using a 3% and 5% discount rate for purposes of comparability with previous studies.
- Consider discounting health effects in monetary and non-monetary terms at a different rate from costs, if there is information available on the change in monetary value of health outcomes over time. However, be aware of the unsettled state of expert opinion on this matter.

Part 2 recommendations: uncertainty and sensitivity analysis

- OHS interventions are subject to uncertainty for a variety of reasons, the key sources of which should be tested through sensitivity analysis.
- Undertake, at a minimum, deterministic univariate, best/worst case scenarios, or multivariate sensitivity analysis for key parameters and/or the functional form of the model.
- Characterize uncertainty about modelling and other methodological assumptions through deterministic sensitivity analysis.
- Make explicit, in deterministic sensitivity analysis, the reasons for choosing alternative parameter values or model specifications.
- Consider undertaking Probabilistic Sensitivity Analysis (PSA) of all important parameters.
- Make explicit, in PSA, the rationale for assigning parameters to specific distributions within the description of methods.
- Present PSA using confidence ellipses and scatter plots on the cost-effectiveness plane, and with cost-effectiveness acceptability curves.
- Consider a Bayesian approach to PSA if the statistical skills and software are available.

Chapter 13

Equity

Anthony J. Culyer and Emile Tompa

Equity in the context of economic evaluations

A basic tenet of economics is that resources are scarce, so it is in the interest of individuals and societies to put them to their best uses. This is the notion underlying allocative efficiency—to get the most for the least. Economic evaluation is a tool to assist with achieving it. Invariably, it requires placing values on both the resources consumed and the consequences their use has produced in order to compare inputs and outputs within and across alternatives. Also inherent in the process is the need to compare and, where appropriate, aggregate costs and consequences across individuals and groups.

Allocative efficiency is a central objective in economic evaluation, but equity is equally important. Equity is commonly considered to be of two main kinds: distributive equity/justice, which refers to the fairness of the allocation of benefits and burdens, and procedural equity/justice, which refers to the fairness and acceptability of decision-making processes (see Box 13.1 for definitions).

Within the broad equity constructs of distributive and procedural justice there are many rival notions. All have it in common that they embody values, so none can be assessed solely on scientific terms. They are also based upon an idea of distancing the balancing of conflicting interests in a way that is detached from personally or institutionally selfish interests. They are intended to inform behaviour or decisions that help answer questions such as: 'how ought management choose between alternatives?', 'should monetary costs and consequences accruing to workers be valued the same as monetary costs and consequences to employers?', 'what is a fair distribution?', 'what is the fairest way to prioritize occupational health and safety (OHS) options (within a workplace, a region, or a jurisdiction)?'. Equity concepts, both distributive and procedural, involve more than one person; they are about relationships and comparisons of people (both individuals and groups). In short, they are about making interpersonal comparisons.

Equity (or its absence) is a characteristic of a society. It is usually treated at the macro- (country, societal) or meso- (system) level, but in some cases it is

Box 13.1 Key efficiency and equity constructs

Allocative efficiency: refers to a situation in which resources are allocated to production processes and the outputs of these processes to consumers so as to maximize the net benefit to society.

Distributive equity/justice: concerns what is just or fair with respect to the allocation of benefits and burdens (consequences and costs) between individuals or groups of individuals. The focus is on outcomes.

Procedural equity/justice: concerns the fairness and transparency by which decisions are made. The focus is on process.

treated at the micro-level, where, perhaps, no more than two people are involved, as for example in physician–patient relationships. In the health economics literature, textbooks such as McGuire *et al.* (1992), Mooney (1992), Dolan and Olsen (2002), Folland *et al.* (2004), and Donaldson *et al.* (2005) focus on macro- and meso-equity issues associated with health care system design and evaluation. Few discuss the central topic of this chapter: the microeconomics of economic evaluation using CEA, CUA and CBA methods. We discuss macro- and meso-level equity, but try also to provide some initial guidance on how best to address equity issues, of whatever kind, in the context of economic evaluations of OHS interventions.

Since equity is a topic in several disciplines, we recommend a few references as a starting point to scoping out a vast literature. For a review of equity from a general philosophical perspective see Plant (1991). For a review of equity from a general economics perspective, see Hausman and McPherson (2006), and for a more specific health-oriented philosophical perspective see Daniels (1985). Williams and Cookson (2000) provide a good review of the equity literature focusing on the macro- and meso-health economics perspective. Wagstaff and van Doorslaer (2000) also provide a review of the health economics perspective, but with a focus on finance and delivery.

Equity and equality

There is an important characteristic that concepts of equity have in common—they all have to do with equality or inequality. Thus, it becomes important to ask the question: equality or inequality of what? Equity does not equate to equality, however. Sometimes one deals with 'just inequalities' and the question is then 'what is the criterion for deciding which inequalities are fair or unfair?' Equity means treating likes alike and unalike appropriately differently. It requires that relevantly similar cases be treated in similar ways and relevantly different cases be treated in appropriately different ways. This brings to the fore two important concepts: horizontal equity and vertical equity. Horizontal equity is the equal treatment of people who are equal in a relevant respect. Vertical equity is the unequal treatment of people who are unequal in a relevant respect (see Box 13.2 for details). It also requires us to be clear about what factors count as relevant respects.

In the context of OHS interventions and the associated costs incurred and consequences produced, equal or unequal treatment for the purpose of fairness or equity amounts to assigning priorities to costs and consequences accordingly. As has been seen in previous chapters, many research studies arbitrarily restrict the categories of cost or consequence considered, for example, by ignoring costs or consequences that fall on workers' families or by attributing an implicitly high weight to positive productivity effects on the bottom line or by minimizing the negative consequences of OHS interventions for companies and their owners. There are probably some implicit social values underlying these biases but, quite

Box 13.2 Horizontal and vertical equity

Horizontal and vertical equity are constructs of fairness often called upon in health care and tax policy. These are two principal areas of social systems where similar treatment of equals and dissimilar treatment of unequals is at the forefront of notions of fairness or justice. In health care, the concern is often the fair distribution of health care services, of the burden (usually on individuals) of financing them or of health itself. In finance policy, it is the fair distribution of tax burdens or, in a labour force context, the fairness of the premiums on employers that often fund the system.

Horizontal equity: the equal treatment of people who are equal in a relevant respect. In health care, the relevant criterion for equality of treatment may be equality of needs, abilities to benefit, or some other aspect that makes individuals equal in their deservedness or entitlement to health care services. In tax policy, the relevant criterion is often equality of incomes.

Vertical equity: is the unequal treatment of people who are unequal in a relevant respect. In health care, individuals may be considered unequal in their deservedness due to differences in need or some other relevant respect. In tax policy, individuals are often treated unequally when their incomes differ (as in progressive taxation).

apart from the unattractiveness of using analytical methods that mask, rather than expose, important equity issues, what might the relevant criteria be for inclusion or exclusion or differential weighting? What criteria correspond to these relevant respects? Drawing on the health care literature, we describe several commonly adopted equity criteria.

One very common criterion is need. In terms of horizontal and vertical equity it requires the equal treatment of people with equal needs and more favourable treatment of people with greater needs. A fundamental challenge with this criterion is that it is far from clear how to define need. It can be defined by ill health, which would suggest that people who are equally ill ought to be treated the same (i.e., receive the same priority in attending to or treating their injury or disease), and those that are sickest ought to receive higher priority. Need might also be defined by risk exposure, in which case people equally at risk of injury, disease, or death ought to be treated the same, and those with greater risk should be given priority.

A key disadvantage of the need criterion is that it appears to assume that all the conditions in question are equally treatable by health care or preventive measures, and that all conditions or hazardous situations are equally costly to remedy. However, this is clearly not always the case. It does not make much sense to provide equal priority for health care services to individuals with equal need if their ability to benefit differs substantially or if the costs of health care provision are vastly different. In the context of OHS interventions, it can hardly be appropriate to require a workplace to provide health care services or preventive measures regardless of effectiveness or cost simply because of equality of need defined by risk exposure or rates of sickness absenteeism. In short, the proportionality requirement implied by the criterion of need (and the share of resources the criterion suggests that each workplace receive) seems arbitrary and, therefore, inequitable.

A second common criterion is deservedness (desert). This criterion requires that people having equal deservedness be treated the same and people with greater deservedness be given higher priority. Aspects of deservedness that proponents of this view often have in mind are lifestyle choices, such as macho workplace behaviours, smoking, drug abuse, poor diet, dangerous sports, careless, and promiscuous sex that increase exposures to deleterious health risks, and the probability of experiencing injury, disease, or death. Lifestyle choices that adversely affect health are grounds for giving individuals that make such choices a low priority. In contrast, individuals with greater deservedness should be given higher priority. Greater deservedness may be based on characteristics such as clean living, higher productivity, more dependent children, or more public service work.

There are two critical concerns with the criterion of deservedness. First, it is difficult to distinguish empirically between lifestyle choices and other factors that bear on health. Secondly, it assumes that lifestyle differences are avoidable, rather than socially conditioned, thus making the people in question culpable for the impact of these differences on their health. In this respect, the criterion comes close to victim-blaming. For example, is it fair to blame (or to discriminate against) a drug-addicted youth for her/his poor health if that youth had parents with similar addictions, and was raised in a deprived and marginalized household? In the workplace setting, is it fair to blame a worker for compromising her/his health following a workplace accident in which the person did not wear the appropriate safety equipment? It might have been that the safety equipment was not provided by management or emphasis was given to expediency, rather than safety, or that it was widely perceived that the general culture of the organization gave safety a very low priority. Even the apparently quantifiable criterion of deservedness based on social contribution is difficult to measure without arbitrariness. Are claimed contributions to be taken at face value? Can one meaningfully separate the productive contributions made in team work? Might not even partial measures of deservingness exacerbate rather than diminish inequity?

A third criterion concerns the resources employed to address equity issues. This criterion is usually presented as a strictly horizontal equity argument. It suggests that, since all people are to be regarded as fundamentally equal, each individual ought to have an equal amount of resources available to address health concerns, and that the per capita distribution ought to be everywhere the same. While the criterion is usually thought of in the context of assigning health care budgets to regional health care providers or commissioning agencies, it is also implicit in claims that certain workplaces, or occupational groups, or industries have an unfair share of OHS resources.

A primary disadvantage of this criterion is that, like the criterion of need, it ignores the productivity of the resources expended to address health concerns. It is difficult to justify an equal expenditure of resources in cases where the capacity to benefit differs. For example, it would seem inappropriate to invest an equal amount of resources in prevention in all workplaces, when in some cases it may be very effective (and low cost) and in others quite ineffective (and high cost). The same issue arises with resources expended for the treatment of health care conditions arising from workplace exposures. What is equitable about expending the same amount regardless of the injured or ill worker's capacity to benefit from it?

This leads to a fourth equity criterion: capacity to benefit. This requires that people with an equal capacity to benefit be given equal treatment and those with greater capacity be given priority. Applied to the workplace, it suggests that people with an equal capacity to benefit health-wise from a workplace intervention ought to be treated the same, and those with higher capacities to benefit ought to be given priority and/or have more resources expended on them.

While the capacity to benefit criterion addresses the concern about the productivity of resources invested in health care and prevention, it so happens that individuals with a relatively greater capacity to benefit generally have better health to begin with (e.g., individuals with higher education and higher income). Hence, the application of this criterion in health care and the workplace context would exacerbate existing health and income/wealth inequalities. This equity criterion is a good example of how there can be fundamental conflicts between different equity criteria.

A fifth criterion on which to base equality is health itself. The objective of this criterion is to achieve the greatest possible equality of health by giving priority to those with relatively poor health. This approach was formalized in Rawl's maximin principle (Rawls 1971), which we discuss in the next section. The equality of health criterion could be implemented by prioritizing interventions based on the level of health of individuals in different work settings (e.g., by giving higher priority to and/or investing more resources in those who are the furthest away from the average health level of the population), or based on the level of health risk exposure in a workplace.

A key disadvantage of the equality of health criterion is that it suggests expending enormous amounts of resources for very sick individuals or those most at risk. However, such interventions may not be very health enhancing and they might well be undertaken at the expense of interventions that would generate much greater health gains for others. This concern is similar to that presented in the equality of need criterion.

A sixth equity criterion is equity of access. In health care it is often framed as equality of access for equal needs. It would entail providing equal access for equal needs and priority access for greater needs. This criterion is perhaps the most frequently encountered type of equity criterion invoked in health care, but could also be applied to OHS interventions. For example, one could allow for equality of access to health and safety training programmes or equality of access for worksites to resources for investment in prevention interventions. Greater need might be defined by productivity or income, and hence priority or faster access to health care and return-to-work services might be given to injured workers on the grounds of their economic productivity or to minimize compensation benefits.

A disadvantage of this criterion is that it might result in high costs if many workers exercise their right to access, yet health gains associated with access may vary substantially. Related to this concern is that health inequalities may persist, and there may remain many untapped gains that could be had at a low cost.

Table 13.1 presents a synopsis of the six equity criteria. The six are not an exhaustive list of possible criteria, but are illustrative of the many and conflicting ways in which equity may be defined. Each has disadvantages and no one is best for all decision contexts. Ultimately, a process in which stakeholders and decision makers participate in the assessment of equity implications of an evaluation might result in the most appropriate choice of equity principle to adopt for a particular situation.

Table 13.1 Summary of equity criteria.

Equity criteria	Horizontal equity interpretation	Vertical equity interpretation	Disadvantages
Proportionality of need (process)	Treat people with equal needs the same	Give priority to people with greater needs	Capacity to benefit may differ for similar needs Cost may differ to address similar needs
Proportionality of deservedness (process)	Treat people with equal deservedness the same	Give priority to people with greater deservedness	Difficult to distinguish between choices and other factors Assumes lifestyle differences are choices Difficult to measure social contributions
Proportionality of expenditures (process)	Provide an equal amount of resources for each person	—	Capacity to benefit may differ across individuals Local price variations result in different resources per person
Proportionality of capacity to benefit (outcomes)	Treat people with equal capacity to benefit the same	Give priority to people with greater capacity to benefit	Can exacerbate existing inequalities since capacity is generally higher for healthier, higher income individuals
Proportionality of health endowment (outcomes)	Treat people with equal health the same	Give priority to those with relatively poor health	Maximin principle suggests expending enormous amount of resources on the worst off Small gains at high cost may be at the expense of large gains at low cost
Proportionality of access (process)	Provide equal access for people with equal needs	Give priority access for people with greater needs	Substantial resources may be expended if access is exercised Capacity to benefit may differ for similar needs Health inequalities may persist Large gains at low costs may remain untapped

Efficiency versus equity

There is a fairly robust tradition in both the economics and the philosophical literatures that casts efficiency and equity in competing roles. While it is undoubtedly true that conflicts can arise, it is helpful to bear in mind two considerations:

◆ the tension between rival equity criteria is greater and often harder to resolve than the tension between equity and efficiency;

◆ the tension between equity and efficiency arises largely because efficiency requires the aggregation of individual consequences, and if this aggregation is undertaken without thought being given to its distributive equity implications, it is highly likely that the efficient alternative will appear inequitable (Culyer 2006).

The tension between rival equity criteria may be hard to resolve, but it can at least be elucidated by identifying and clarifying the criteria under consideration. In the context of a specific evaluation, if there is a concern about the relevant criteria to be considered, then offering stakeholders and decision makers a list of possibilities as presented in Table 13.1 may be a useful point of departure.

The apparent tension between efficiency and distributive equity can be illustrated by an example from health technology assessment. A typical evaluation would consider the health consequences of alternative treatment options measured in Quality-Adjusted Life-Years (QALYs). The objective may be specified as selecting the technology with the highest incremental cost–utility ratio from a set of possible options. Total health consequences would be measured as the net present value of a discounted stream of future QALYs and added across the individuals who are predicted to benefit. Simple addition within and across individuals assumes that the social value of an additional QALY is the same, regardless of who receives it and how many any one individual receives. Essentially, all QALYs are given equal weight.

Should it turn out that QALYs are thought to be of different value depending on who receives them and/or how many are received by any one individual, then the efficient alternative might be in conflict with the relevant equity criterion. The conflict disappears if appropriate weights are attached to QALYs instead of assuming equal value. Weights might be based on generic characteristics of recipients, such as age, gender, and number of QALYs received (we discuss equity weights in greater detail later in the chapter). Alternatively, the efficiency analysis based on the assumption of equal value of QALYs could be explicitly presented as provisional, with the ultimate decision to be taken after a decision-making body gives due consideration to the equity implications of alternatives in addition to the provisional efficiency analysis. The key point is that both efficiency and equity must be considered in tandem, with neither trumping the other.

Perhaps the principal lesson from this brief review of equity criteria is to emphasize the importance of being clear about the underlying equity principles being invoked when assessing the distributive equity of alternatives. As is apparent in the above descriptions there are multiple concepts of equity, some of which are mutually compatible and others which are not. Many discussions of equity are typically fraught with generalized slogans and particular interest groups will tend to select those that most favour their own interests. In order to enhance the clarity of analyses of the equity implications within the context of economic evaluations, we suggest considering, consulting and reporting the answers to the following questions:

- What are the appropriate relevant respects (criteria) to be borne in mind in the situation at hand?

- Are the equity criteria under consideration appropriately distanced from the particular interests likely to be affected by the intervention?

- Are the equity criteria addressing horizontal or vertical equity?

- Are the equity criteria addressing process such as access or exposure (procedural justice) or outcome/consequences such as better health (distributive justice)?

Equity constructs

In what follows, we review several well-known equity constructs found in the literature. Some have been considered in the economics literature, and specifically in health economics, whereas others come from other disciplines. Some approaches provide guidance on how to embody equity in a decision-making algorithm, as through the use of weights to adjust health or utility values based on the characteristics of recipients. Others provide guidance on how equity concerns can be incorporated alongside evidence into the decision-making process itself in order to afford an opportunity for decision makers to delve more deeply by considering the individuals that are likely to gain or lose from an intervention and the nature of their gains or losses. Decision makers may also consider how best to manage the introduction of a worthwhile intervention that has both gains and uncompensated losses in light of equity concerns. Our emphasis is on providing appropriate information to decision makers rather than deciding precisely how equity is to be embodied in the analysis.

The fair innings approach

Williams' (1997) fair innings approach was developed in the context of the UK's National Health Service (NHS) to address issues of distributive equity, specifically as they related to vertical equity. The approach assumes that one of the objectives of the NHS is to reduce inequalities in people's lifetime experience of health. Age matters in two respects. First, it affects people's capacity to benefit and, therefore, places older people at a general disadvantage if another objective is to maximize the (unweighted) benefits of health care. Secondly, older people are more likely to have had fair innings in terms of experiencing many years of healthy life and this places them at a lower priority based on the notion of minimizing differences in lifetime health. Williams argued that it would be equitable to provide small benefits to young people even if, in so doing, the elderly were denied large benefits, provided that the young recipients had a low probability of achieving a fair innings. The approach does not necessitate young people having absolute priority for benefits compared with older people. Rather, it simply means that their health benefits are given greater weight. Applied to economic evaluative methods, the fair innings approach suggests that generic characteristic be used to weight benefits (and possibly costs) differently. Age would be the principal characteristic to consider, though other characteristics might also be used in the developing weights. In all cases, the following three factors should be considered:

- Is the ethical argument for weighting benefits differently based on a recipient's characteristics acceptable in the context of the given evaluation?

- Is there an acceptable method for identifying or developing appropriate weights?

- Are the issues involved best addressed by weighting benefits or through a deliberative approach that would allow for additional evidence to be considered in the decision-making process?

The World Health Organization developed a weighting system based on age for use with a health outcome measure known as Disability-Adjusted Life-Years (DALYs) to measure the global burden of disease (Murray and Lopez 1996b). DALYs measure the health gap due to injury, disease and premature mortality based on a gold standard of a full and healthy life of 80 years for men and 82.5 years for women. Weights were developed for DALYs based on the notion that years of healthy life in early adulthood are worth the most to society. DALYs during the early years of life from birth are given lesser weight, but increase substantially in the years to early adulthood and decline gradually thereafter into old age.

Justice as fairness

Rawls (1971) developed a theory of equity that has been particularly influential for health economists, even though he explicitly excluded health and health care in his analysis of justice as fairness. Rawls proposed a hypothetical situation for assessing equity issues in which individuals making decisions are shrouded by a 'veil of ignorance', such that they have no knowledge about their own personal circumstances or position in society. Such a veil provides a distance between self interest and considerations of equity. Rawls conjectured that such an approach would result in an agreement on two basic principles of fairness:

◆ basic liberties (such as the right to vote, freedom of speech, and the right to own property) ought to be both equally distributed and as complete as is consistent with equality;

◆ primary goods (such as basic liberties, income and wealth, position of responsibility, and respect) should be distributed such that only inequalities that were to the benefit of the least advantaged people would be permitted. This criterion is known as the maximin principle.

Primary goods include attributes essentially determined by the interactions in human societies, but not 'natural goods', such as health. Primary goods are a means to an end, a means to attaining welfare. Rawls excluded health from the list of primary goods because health is an end in itself, because it is determined largely by nature, and because he felt that the application of the maximin principle to health could lead to large amounts of health care resources being devoted to the health of people who would gain little from it, possibly at the expense of driving others into poverty.

Equity and capabilities

Sen (1980, 1993) argued that non-utility characteristics often provide better grounds for assessing the equity implications of alternative social states than utility and welfare. According to Sen, a particularly important class of non-utility information is people's basic capabilities. These capabilities are ones that enable people to engage in activities that are important to them, such as working, using leisure time, community involvement, and living a healthy life. Equity concerns should thus focus on the distribution of basic capabilities. The approach suggests that equity is about moving society towards a more equal distribution of capabilities. Sen suggested that many basic capabilities can be measured as levels of functioning. This is certainly true for health.

The basic capabilities approach is extra-welfarist in that it goes beyond the evaluation of human welfare and its distribution in terms of individual utilities.

The approach does not provide an algorithm. Its value lies in the framework it provides for thinking about equity issues. It leaves a good deal to the discretion of analysts, such as determining what counts as basic capabilities in health and in a workplace context, how they are to be measured and weighted. One approach for the economic analyst might be to create a process for reasoned agreement with stakeholders, bearing in mind the specific decision context.

The rule of rescue

The rule of rescue approach to equity consists of an injunction to rescue identifiable individuals in immediate peril, regardless of cost. The plausibility of the rule is well-expressed in the following quote (Jonsen 1996, cited by Cookson *et al.* 2007):

> Our moral response to the imminence of death demands that we rescue the doomed. We throw a rope to the drowning, rush into burning buildings to snatch the entrapped, dispatch teams to search for the snowbound. This rescue morality spills over into medical care, where our ropes are artificial hearts, our rush is the mobile critical care unit, our teams are the transplant services.

The appeal of the rule lies in the heroics expressed in the rescue process. The downside is that though an intervention may rescue people facing imminent death, it may give them only a small increment in extra life. Furthermore, the cost of funding the rescue technology may divert resources away from other activities that provide substantially greater benefits to others. Essentially, the rule of rescue focuses on the benefit to one group (whose identities are usually known) and ignores the cost to others (who are probably anonymous potential beneficiaries of forgone opportunities). There is an implicit interpersonal comparison, which values the benefits of one group over those of another. Concern for identifiable individuals in immediate peril unambiguously implies less concern for unidentifiable individuals in future peril. Such discrimination, when it is seen for what it is, seems intuitively unpalatable. Although it is based on a natural human expression of good will, it entails gross inconsistency in the way it treats the value of resources (Cookson *et al.* 2007). The approach is not the same as having a concern for the severity of a current health condition or risk exposure in a working environment. Rather, it would suggest providing increases in safety of a value that need not be compared with its cost in order to favour identified individuals at the expense of the unidentified.

Libertarianism

Some procedural approaches operate at a very broad level. Libertarianism in its classical forms (e.g., Locke 1967) or its contemporary version (e.g., Alchian 1965;

Nozick 1974) accords a minimal role to the state, based on the premise that there is little justification for any regulation beyond that required to operate a system of exchangeable private property rights. There is no scope for agencies to promote or regulate efficiency, equity or health and safety. No individual's right, small or large, should ever be sacrificed for any other end, including the rights of other. This approach is tantamount to denying the legitimacy of any concept of equity, unless outcomes are automatically defined as equitable if they are a product of an equitable process which, according to libertarianism, would exist in a market uncluttered by regulation. The pure form of libertarianism plainly implies that allocative decision-making tools such as economic evaluation are not libertarian. However, provided that the stakeholders in any given practical situation in which an economic evaluation is being planned can agree that the existing rights and entitlements of stakeholders are satisfactory, it is possible that a case can be made for a consultative process that would determine the methods to be used to choose the optimal set of health and safety interventions and how evidence, and what kind of evidence, would be incorporated into the process.

Accountability for reasonableness

A much less extreme approach than libertarianism is that of 'accountability for reasonableness' (Daniels and Sabin 1998; Daniels 2000). This approach incorporates the fact that there is often reasonable disagreement about relevant equity criteria. The approach provides some principles of a legitimate and fair process for making decisions without needing to specify any specific outcome. Key elements of a fair process include transparency about the grounds for decisions, appeals to rationales that all can accept as relevant to decision making, and procedures for revising decisions in light of challenges to them. Together, these principles ensure accountability for reasonableness. Box 13.3 provides an example of an application of this approach.

Deliberative processes

A deliberative process is characterized by a careful, deliberate consideration and discussion of the advantages and disadvantages of various options in an effort to assist people with making a decision (Hajer and Wagenaar 2003). A deliberative process is used to elicit and combine various types of evidence. A deliberative process integrates scientific analysis and social context with stakeholder or lay public views elicited through consultation and participation. However, a deliberative process is different from a consultative process in that it requires participation rather than simply consultation (see Box 13.4 for an example of a consultative process that was not a deliberative process).

Box 13.3 Application of accountability for reasonableness

Accountability for reasonableness has been adopted by the National Institute for Health and Clinical Excellence (NICE) in the UK. NICE describes accountability for reasonableness as follows (NICE 2007, p. 13): 'For decision makers to be accountable for their reasonableness, the processes they use to make their decisions must have four characteristics: publicity, relevance, challenge and revision, and regulation.'

Publicity: both the decisions made about limits on the allocation of resources, and the grounds for reaching them, must be made public.

Relevance: the grounds for reaching decisions must be ones that fair-minded people would agree are relevant in the particular context.

Challenge and revision: there must be opportunities for challenging decisions that are unreasonable, that are reached through improper procedures, or that exceed the proper powers of the decision makers. There must be mechanisms for resolving disputes and transparent systems available for revising decisions when more evidence becomes available.

Regulation: there should be either voluntary or public regulation of the decision-making process to ensure that it possesses all three of the above characteristics.

Box 13.4 Example of a consultative process

The Oregon priority-setting exercise for health care interventions initiated in 1989 is a well-known example of a consultative process. The exercise entailed 47 community meetings, 12 public hearings and 54 panel meetings with health care providers. The information from these meetings was provided to the Oregon Health Services Commission to inform the prioritization of health care procedures (Garland 1992). Thus, many individuals and groups were consulted, but relatively few participated in the discussions where the data and evidence collected was synthesized and integrated to develop the final prioritization.

Employing a deliberative process increases the likelihood of achieving a sound and acceptable decision (Daniels 2000). If properly executed it will be more comprehensive in the relevant issues embraced, more consistent in the way they are embraced and more engaging of the people affected by the outcome than a closed-door or ad hoc process (Culyer and Lomas 2006).

The following conditions are hypothesized to be those under which a deliberative process is most likely to be warranted:

- evidence from more than one expert discipline is involved;
- evidence from more than one profession is involved;
- stakeholders have conflicting interests;
- there are technical disputes to resolve;
- evidence may be scientifically controversial;
- evidence gathered in one context is to be applied in another;
- costs and consequences extend beyond the conventional boundaries of business planning;
- there is substantial uncertainty about key values and risks, which needs to be assessed and weighed;
- there are social and personal values not taken into consideration in the scientific analyses;
- there are issues of equity involved;
- there are issues of implementability and operational feasibility;
- a wide public and professional ownership is desired.

As is apparent, equity is one of the items on the list, and it is often one of the most important and intractable factors under consideration. A deliberative process is particularly useful when equity is a central concern in a decision because of the uncertainty surrounding the appropriate equity criterion to adopt, the general absence of quantitative data to inform equity issues, and the uncertainty about how to trade off equity against other considerations such as efficiency, implementability and manageability.

Equity and incidence

A matter that may have considerable implications for judgments about equity is the divergence between the initial and final incidence of costs and benefits. The most common application of the theory of incidence in economics is in the field of taxation, where the initial incidence of a tax change is compared with its final incidence or burden after all market adjustments in response to the change have been completed.

As an example, consider the kind of effects that might follow the adoption of a costly new intervention to enhance worker safety. The initial incidence of costs will reside with the firm as new equipment is acquired, old equipment modified, new training schemes deployed and new management structures created. However, in the medium to long term the combination of a safer working environment, and shifts of the skill mix and other substitutions may cause wages to decrease since, all else being equal, a safer environment will generally result in a lower wage (higher wages normally compensating to some extent for higher risks). The effects on the production side may affect overall marginal costs and generate a change in the price of the products produced, which in turn may generate a change in the amount demanded in any time period. It is possible that what was initially a cost to the firm turns out to be no burden at all, with the costs falling on consumers, or workers, or both via higher prices and lower wages. However, the working environment will still be safer than before the intervention, which is of benefit to workers. Moreover, if greater safety has positive productivity effects, it may translate into an increase in wages and profits.

The implications for assessing the equity aspects of OHS interventions should be apparent: if it is possible for the initial incidence of the costs or benefits of any change to be shifted to others, then any assessment of the equity of the change that fails to account for this would be flawed. How significant such effects are is an empirical matter. Whether it is worth modelling these shifts to estimate their magnitude will be a judgment that should be based on factors such as:

- how far reaching the intervention is in terms of the number of workers and firms affected—the greater the scope of the intervention, the more likely it is that incidence will be shifted in ways that might affect judgments of equity;

- the size of the firm level intervention in terms of cost, health and productivity effects—a modest intervention will generate smaller shifts;

- the competitiveness of the labour and product markets in question—less competitive labour and product markets will have smaller elasticities, and hence lesser responses;

- the speed of implementation of the intervention—the costs of slow or gradual implementation tend to be lower than fast implementation and shifting of burdens will take place over a longer period of time;

- the effectiveness of the intervention—a less effective intervention will generate less scope for shifting.

Recommendations

- Identify the relevant stakeholder groups who may gain or lose from an intervention and provide an analysis of the gains and losses by group.
- Ensure, so far as possible, that the idea of equity is distanced from the self-interest of any participating stakeholder group.
- Determine whether the equity issues are horizontal, vertical or a mixture of both.
- Clarify the relevant respect(s) or criteria in terms of which individuals and groups are to be differentiated.
- Decide whether the process of decision making or of subsequent roll-out of the intervention is itself a part of the equitable solution.
- Consider whether equity is better treated in an algorithmic fashion (e.g., by weighting various elements of a calculated cost-effectiveness ratio) or by consultation/deliberation of some sort.
- Consider differential weights for costs and consequences accruing to different individuals and groups. Be clear about their calibration and justification.
- Explore the possibility of determining equity weights through sampling relevant sections of the population.
- Consider whether, should a consultative route be followed, it be merely consultative or also deliberative.
- Be on guard for special pleading masquerading as the rule of rescue.
- Consider, where appropriate, adjusting for the difference between the initial and the final incidence of costs and consequences.

Part 3

Conclusions

Chapter 14

Suggestions for a reference case

Emile Tompa, Anthony J.Culyer, and Roman
Dolinschi

Introduction

A key feature of both Gold *et al* (1996) and NICE (2004) is their provision of
methodological guidance and best practice in the form of a reference case. The
purpose of a reference case is to ensure that methods are based on sound economics and to help ensure that these soundly-based principles are consistently
applied in economic evaluations, regardless of the intervention or the sector in
which the evaluation is undertaken. The primary benefit of standardization is
that it makes the results from different studies more readily comparable.
Having a reference case does not preclude analysts undertaking other types of
analysis or supplementing the guidance embodied in the reference case in
other ways. However, departures from the reference case should be justified on
the basis of potential shortcomings of the reference case for a specific context.

In this chapter we synthesize the summaries, conclusions, challenges, and
recommendations from the preceding chapters to formulate a reference case
for economic evaluations in occupational health and safety (OHS). We think
it is worth trying to build such a professional scientific consensus, and our
prescriptions are intended to serve as a starting point. Our proposed reference
case provides a minimal set of criteria for planning, assembling, and reporting
economic evaluations of OHS interventions.

A reference case for OHS evaluations should permit all relevant perspectives, objectives, and trade-offs to be taken into account, so that the informational needs of workplace parties and of the wider OHS community can be
appropriately addressed. It should enable the scope of the analysis, including
its perspective, to be selected according to the values and intentions of the
stakeholders on whose behalf the study is done. It should also include a broad
perspective, such that all significant costs and consequences, as well as their
distribution, are taken into consideration, and a view given as to the general
social desirability of an intervention, as well as a view from the perspective of
more particular interested parties.

An essential feature of a sound economic evaluation in any domain is the full and explicit reporting of the key structural elements of an analysis, the sources of evidence and the values embodied in the interpretation of findings. The list of ten methodological shortcomings presented in Chapter 3 and the checklist provided in Chapter 4 might be used in conjunction with our reference case prescriptions in this chapter to assist researchers with ensuring that the desirable aspects of a high quality economic evaluation are included and reported in an analysis. Given the complexity and diversity of OHS systems in different jurisdictions, good reporting practice suggests that it is also important to describe the policy environment, key stakeholders, and behavioural incentives created by the OHS system where the study was undertaken. For additional guidance on the presentation and reporting of economic evaluations, we refer readers to Drummond *et al.* (2005, pp. 323–364) and Gold *et al.* (1996, pp. 276–303).

Framework principles

Three ethical principles serve as a common basis for OHS interventions. These provide the foundation for evaluations and are the starting point for our reference case. The first principle makes explicit the purpose of OHS interventions.

> 1) The prime objective of health and safety interventions is to enhance the expected health-related welfare of individuals in the workplace.

Supplementary objectives might also be included in an economic evaluation of an OHS intervention, but this ought to be the primary one. This principle is plainly an ethical statement. It is essentially the same as that which underpins welfare economics in general. It is outlined in Chapters 2 and 5, which make a strong case for focusing on a wide range of human outcomes, rather than merely those that are financial. However, whether human or financial outcomes are more important is an issue of perspective, which brings us to the second principle.

> 2) The perspective of particular evaluative studies will be determined in conjunction with relevant stakeholders and supplemented where necessary by analyses that incorporate significant external effects.

The perspective suggested by this principle may be narrower than the societal perspective (depending on the choices made by stakeholders), but it will be different from and broader than the narrow focus on the business bottom line. This principle is meant to allow for both the pragmatist's concern, such as the bottom line, and the wider interests of other stakeholders. There is a strong case to be made for flexibility in the choice of perspective, since studies may reasonably take different views on the grounds that responsibility for managing resources varies from one situation to another. Common to all OHS evaluations is a focus on those working in the workplaces and likely to participate in, benefit from, or incur costs as a result of the interventions. Where the emphasis should lie in any particular study will be a matter for prior determination by researchers working with research commissioners. Since costs and consequences may be distributed across multiple stakeholders, issues of distributive equity may come to the fore and warrant explicit consideration. This brings us to the third principle.

> 3) Economic evaluations should, in addition to considering efficiency, identify potential equity issues of significance in conjunction with stakeholders and always present results in a way that reveals how the incidence of costs and benefits falls both immediately and after any predictable market adjustments have been made.

The distribution of costs and benefits is important not only so that matters of equity can be addressed, but also in order to facilitate thinking about how an intervention might best be implemented. For example, a costly workplace intervention whose benefit falls entirely on workers and their families in the form of health, and which has no productivity impact, may be amply justified in social terms, but may not be in any individual employer's interest to implement. Such an intervention would require subsidization or legislation to put into effect. Consideration of short- and long-term incidence is also important, since in some cases costs may initially appear to be borne by employers, but over time may be passed on to consumers in the form of higher prices and/or to workers in the form of lower wages.

In what follows we present a summary of the key messages from each specific topic chapter followed by recommendations for good practice. Each recommendation is labelled with either the letter 'R' to refer to a recommendation required for the reference case, or the letter 'G' for a recommendation provided as guidance, but not considered essential for good practice.

Study design

The presence of many factors to be considered when choosing a study design implies that there is no universal design hierarchy to guide the economist and the research team. In general, most evaluations require a synthesis of data from two or more sources. Our general advice is:

- Choose the study design that best ensures that an estimate of net outcomes is both internally and externally valid. **R**
- Be explicit in the research report about the reasons for the choice of study design. **R**

- Consider an experimental design. This design is generally preferred for its internal validity, particularly if issues of external validity can be adequately addressed through synthesis. **G**

- Consider as an alternative to an experimental design, a quasi-experimental design with features enhancing internal validity, such as matched contemporaneous control groups, data collection at multiple points in time pre- and post-intervention, and statistical adjustments. Designs with these features are strong alternatives to experimental designs and under some circumstances represent the preferred approaches. **G**

- Avoid, if possible, case-control studies and before–after designs. These designs introduce severe threats to internal validity of the estimated intervention effect, and are rarely satisfactory as a primary source of evidence for economic evaluations. **G**

Kind of analysis and decision rule

Economic models pose an optimization problem and provide decision rules that prescribe how to use scarce resources optimally. An objective function is postulated along with various constraints based on a given perspective. The solution to the constrained optimization problem identifies how best to use scarce resources.

In practice, it is not always easy to identify the objective, the constraints, or the costs. The answers will certainly depend on who is making the decision, which in turn determines the perspective. Theory can make clear the kind of factors that ought to be considered and thereby identify the kinds of information that should inform the decision maker. Consultation with stakeholders can also help in this process.

Decisions always involve trade-offs. Different ways of describing these trade-offs have given rise to different kinds of economic evaluation [cost–benefit analysis (CBA), cost-effectiveness analysis (CEA), cost–utility analysis (CUA), etc.]. Each involves costs usually measured in monetary terms; the key difference between them lies in how health and other consequences or outcomes are measured. Choosing the appropriate kind of economic evaluation to use in OHS can be a challenge because of the multiple stakeholders involved. A key consideration is the trade-off that matters most to the decision maker.

Our framework principles identified health maximization as the primary objective. This does not, however, preclude the consideration of other objectives alongside it, such as profit maximization (i.e., consideration of financial outcomes). Our general advice is:

- Use one or more appropriate comparator(s) in an economic evaluation and be explicit about what they are. **R**

- For CBA, use the efficiency decision rule: 'adopt interventions having a positive incremental net present value'. **R**

- For CEA and CUA, use the efficiency decision rule: 'adopt interventions where the extra cost is less than the value of the extra outcome (i.e., $\lambda \Delta E - \Delta C > 0$)'. **R**

- Ensure that the choice of the kind of economic evaluation reflects what the decision maker feels is of most importance in terms of outcomes and her/his objectives for the programme. **R**

- Be transparent about the reasons for selecting a particular kind of economic analysis, the outcome of focus, and the accompanying decision rule. **R**

- Do not assume that the efficiency decision rules are dominant over other considerations such as the equity of the distribution of costs and consequences and the feasibility of implementation. **R**

- Be explicit about the perspective from which the study is done and the level of decision making (e.g., firm, system, societal). **R**

- Be transparent about areas of uncertainty and assumptions, so that the decision maker can place results in her/his own context. **R**

- Indicate key data that are judged to have been measured well and those judged to have been measured poorly, and avoid combining both types into a single number. **G**

- Consider trade-offs when presenting options and focus on opportunity costs (e.g., what would be forgone in order to pay for the current candidate programme). **G**

- Compare results with those of other similar studies where these exist. **G**

- Explicitly consider the issues raised for regulation and/or subsidy when societal considerations indicate the net desirability of an intervention, but the organization sees only net costs. **G**

Costs

Economic costs are not always easily identified by the inspection of accounts. The underlying idea of a cost is that it is the most valued alternative use of a resource (i.e., the opportunity cost). Costs will always be contingent on the perspective of a study and on the nature of the decision.

Input resources specific to the intervention should be treated as costs and all other resource implications (values created and resources saved) should be classified as consequences along with the key outcome(s) of interest. Monetized consequences may be positive or negative and would be included in the NPV in a CBA, or in the numerator of the ratio in a CEA or CUA.

An issue that can cause confusion is the treatment of 'indirect costs'. There is less than complete agreement about what constitutes direct or indirect and we suggest, rather than labelling them as indirect, simply identifying them explicitly by name. The term 'indirect costs' often refers to external costs (i.e., costs that fall on individuals and others that are not party to the decision) and changes in productivity directly due to the decision. Two types of productivity change should be distinguished:

◆ temporary productivity effects attributable to down time, while new equipment is installed, and time spent learning to use a new machine or to undertake a new process;

◆ long-term productivity effects directly related to the intervention or mediated through health improvements.

The former are legitimate costs of implementing an intervention, while the latter are consequences of the intervention, and may be positive or negative. If they are negative, it is tempting to regard them as costs whereas it is better to count them as consequences (ones whose value ought to be deducted from the positive benefits). Our general advice is:

◆ Make the analytic and measurement time frame explicit. **R**

◆ Ensure that costs are reasonable approximations to opportunity costs, given the perspective. **R**

◆ Use incremental rather than total or average costs. **R**

◆ Consider the decision context (e.g., timing and speed of introduction, and duration of the intervention) and the ways in which that might affect costs. **G**

◆ Consider including costs of the intervention occurring beyond the measurement time frame and be explicit about how they are formulated. **G**

◆ Distinguish, in the detailed reporting, between productivity costs (inputs to the intervention such as worker time for training and down time for new equipment installation) and productivity consequences (e.g., increases in productivity and/or product quality directly due to the intervention or mediated through health). **G**

◆ Present disaggregated costs by component and stakeholder in addition to a summary measure. **R**

◆ Present time losses and wage rates separately. **G**

◆ Adjust costs for inflation so that all estimates are in constant prices (see also the recommendations under time preference). **R**

◆ Discount costs using an appropriate discount rate (see also the recommendations under time preference). **R**

◆ Test the impact of various assumptions about costs through sensitivity analysis (see also the recommendations under uncertainty). **R**

Consequences

Given the complexity of OHS systems, an intervention may result in changes in activity across different types of disability insurance programmes. Therefore, it is important for researchers evaluating an intervention to look at a broad range of insurance and social programmes available to workers and employers to identify the full extent of consequences, and their distribution across stakeholders.

Depending on the way in which the health outcome measure is constructed, the productivity consequences of health improvements may or may not be included in it. If they are not, productivity changes can be measured as a distinct consequence of the intervention. One must be conscious of how these consequences are captured in order to avoid double counting or inadvertently excluding them.

Incorporating monetary measures of productivity into economic evaluations will, all else being equal, result in larger estimates of value in programmes directed at the working population and, within working populations, at those earning higher incomes. There are often distributional issues that might not be immediately apparent, but which should be explicitly drawn out by the analyst. Our general advice is:

◆ Be alert to the possibility that occupational injury and disease costs may be shifted from one programme/stakeholder to another. **R**

◆ Be explicit about the range of costs that arise from occupational injury and disease, which represent possible benefits if averted. **R**

◆ Measure, when possible, the value of health separately from averted productivity costs. **G**

◆ Consider the friction cost approach if measuring averted productivity costs separately from health. **G**

◆ Be alert to the risk of double counting productivity consequences in measures of health effects or inadvertently not including them at all. **G**

◆ Be explicit, when valuing health and productivity consequences in monetary terms, about the method used to value them (human capital, revealed-preference, or stated-preference) and use it consistently, bearing in mind the very significant differences in results that each can give. **R**

◆ Be alert to the risk of biasing measures of gain or loss by use of techniques that reflect ability to pay. **G**

- Be alert to the possibility of productivity losses through presenteeism, as well as absenteeism. **G**
- Consider including consequences of the intervention occurring beyond the measurement time frame and be explicit about how they are formulated. **G**
- Present disaggregated consequences by category for each stakeholder separately in addition to the summary measure. **G**
- Adjust monetary consequences for inflation so that all estimates are in constant prices (see also the recommendations under time preference). **R**
- Discount monetary and non-monetary consequences using an appropriate discount rate (see also the recommendations under time preference). **R**
- Test the impact of various assumptions about consequences through sensitivity analysis (see also the recommendations under uncertainty). **R**
- Undertake conversion of specific outcome measures to general ones, or intermediate to final, on the basis of the best empirical knowledge available about the relationship between them (either causal or simply an association), and never leave details of the conversion implicit and undiscussed. **G**
- Consider using utility measures of health changes associated with OHS interventions rather than conventional morbidity or mortality data, or conventional workplace participation data. **G**

Time preference

The differential timing of resource flows for alternative interventions can only be meaningfully compared by translating them to a common point in time, usually the present or the start date of the intervention. Adjustment for inflation is done for reasons different from those for adjustment for time preference, although in some cases the rate used to discount flows may include both time preference and inflation in one value. It is preferable to address the issues of inflation and time preference separately if possible, in order to allow for the use of different rates of time preference for the purpose of sensitivity analysis. Our general advice is:

- Adjust costs and monetary consequences occurring over multiple years for inflation. **R**
- As a separate exercise, discount costs and monetary consequences occurring over multiple years to the start of the intervention or the time of decision to intervene. **R**
- Discount non-monetary consequences occurring over multiple years to the start of the intervention or the time of decision to intervene. **R**

- Use a discount rate that is relevant to the decision maker. **R**
- Consider using a 3% and 5% discount rate for purposes of comparability with previous studies. **G**
- Consider discounting health effects in monetary and non-monetary terms at a different rate from costs, if there is information available on the change in monetary value of health outcomes over time. However, be aware of the unsettled state of expert opinion on this matter. **G**

Uncertainty

OHS interventions are subject to uncertainty for a variety of reasons, the key sources of which should be tested through sensitivity analysis. There are several reasons why uncertainty in economic evaluations should be characterized expressly and accurately. Characterizing uncertainty can provide insight into the robustness of results under alternative scenarios; reveal additional data requirements before an intervention is widely adopted; inform future research directions; and influence the timing of a reappraisal of an evaluation in anticipation of additional evidence becoming available. Our general advice is:

- Undertake, at a minimum, deterministic univariate, best/worst case scenarios, or multivariate sensitivity analysis for key parameters and/or the functional form of the model. **R**
- Characterize uncertainty about modelling and other methodological assumptions through deterministic sensitivity analysis. **G**
- Make explicit, in deterministic sensitivity analysis, the reasons for choosing alternative parameter values or model specifications. **R**
- Consider undertaking Probabilistic Sensitivity Analysis (PSA) of all important parameters. **G**
- Make explicit, in PSA, the rationale for assigning parameters to specific distributions within the description of methods. **G**
- Present PSA using confidence ellipses and scatter plots on the cost-effectiveness plane, and with cost-effectiveness acceptability curves. **G**
- Consider a Bayesian approach to PSA if the statistical skills and software are available. **G**

Equity in economic evaluation

All equity constructs embody values, so none can be assessed solely on scientific terms. They are also based upon an idea of balancing the conflicting interests in a way that is detached from personally or institutionally selfish interests.

There is an important characteristic that equity concepts have in common: they all have to do with equality or inequality. Equity thus means treating likes alike and unalikes appropriately differently. It requires that relevant similar cases be treated in similar ways, and relevant different cases be treated in appropriately different ways. It therefore requires clarity about what factors count as relevant respects. Our general advice is:

- Identify the relevant stakeholder groups who may gain or lose from an intervention, and provide an analysis of the gains and losses by group. **R**

- Ensure, so far as possible, that the idea of equity is distanced from the self-interest of any participating stakeholder group. **R**

- Determine whether the equity issues are horizontal, vertical, or a mixture of both. **G**

- Clarify the relevant respect(s) or criteria in terms of which individuals and groups are to be differentiated. **G**

- Decide whether the process of decision making or of subsequent roll-out of the intervention is itself a part of the equitable solution. **G**

- Consider whether equity is better treated in an algorithmic fashion (e.g., by weighting various elements of a calculated cost-effectiveness ratio) or by consultation/deliberation of some sort. **G**

- Consider differential weights for costs and consequences accruing to different individuals and groups and be clear about their calibration and justification. **G**

- Explore the possibility of determining equity weights through sampling relevant sections of the population. **G**

- Consider whether, should a consultative route be followed, it be merely consultative or also deliberative. **G**

- Be on guard for special pleading masquerading as the rule of rescue. **G**

- Consider, where appropriate, adjusting for the difference between the initial and the final incidence of costs and consequences. **G**

Glossary

Absenteeism workers' unscheduled absences from the workplace.

Accountability for reasonableness a decision-making procedure that enables agreement on what is a legitimate and fair way of making decisions, without specifying any necessary specific outcome. Key elements involve transparency about the grounds for decisions, appeals to rationales that all can accept as relevant and fair, and procedures for revising decisions in light of challenges to them.

Adverse selection an insurance-related process in which individuals with a risk level known to them that differs from the risk level used in premium setting self-select into or out of insurance, resulting in a higher average population risk than initially assumed by the insurer. For example, if members of subsets of the population believe they have different probabilities of illness from those on which insurance premiums are set, then people with low perceived probabilities may not buy insurance and those with high perceptions may eagerly seize the opportunity. If this happens, insurers end up with clients who are likely to prove costlier than expected.

Aetiology the study of the causes of disease.

Agency relationship the relationship between an agent (q.v.) and a principal (q.v.).

Agent an actor in an economic system who acts of behalf of another (the principal, q.v.). Classically, a doctor acting on behalf of a patient.

Allocative efficiency a situation in which resources are allocated to production processes and the outputs of these processes to consumers so as to maximize the net benefit to society. Pareto efficiency (q.v.) is a specific form of it.

Amortization the process through which a debt is gradually reduced over time by periodic payments sufficient to pay current interest and to eliminate the principal at maturity.

Ascertainment bias a form of selection bias. For example, women taking an oral contraceptive tend to have more frequent cervical smears than women who are not and so are more likely to have cervical cancer diagnosed. Thus, in a case-control study (q.v.) that compared women with cervical cancer with a control group, at least part of any higher pill consumption rates amongst the former group may be due to this effect. Also called 'detection bias'.

Asymmetry of information a situation in which one individual or group possesses knowledge that another group, with which it is dealing, does not.

Attrition the exclusion or drop-out of individuals for a particular reason after assignment to the intervention or control.

Base year the year or date at which an index takes the value 100.

Bayesian approach a statistical way of revising beliefs about probabilities or the value of parameters as new information is obtained. The revised probabilities are known as a 'posterior distribution of probabilities'.

Before–after study a study in which outcomes are measured at one point in time before an intervention is implemented and compared with outcomes measured at another later point in time. Also called a 'pre–post study'.

Between-individual variability a variability of outcome due to the effects of identifiable subgroups of individuals who differ by age, sex, job, firm characteristics, regulatory environment, and other covariates, or who differ by unmeasured differences.

Bias any systematic difference between the empirical results of an analysis and the true facts of the case. In non-statistical areas it is any distorting influence that might systematically lead to wrong or misleading results. For example, a search of the English language literature on a subject might lead one to ignore all Chinese contributions and to conclude something wrong. Research sponsorship (whether by commercial or non-commercial sponsors) can lead to pressure on researchers to produce particular results or suppress unwanted results. Bias, fraud apart, is broadly of three kinds: informational (as when there are systematic coding errors); selection (as when there are systematic distortions in the ways which experimental subjects are selected) and confounding (as when some determinants are not controlled for).

Bivariate sensitivity analysis a form of sensitivity analysis (q.v.) in which two parameters (q.v.) are varied at a time.

Blinding an experimental arrangement in which either the subjects or the experimenters do not know whether a subject has been allocated to the experimental or the control (q.v.) arm of the trial. When both groups are blind it is described as a 'double blind' trial.

Blocked randomization in blocked randomization, subjects are allocated to groups and then randomly allocated to intervention or control.

Budget constraint a limit on expenditure imposed by a cash-limited budget that cannot be exceeded in any given period of time.

Burden of disease a measure of the total morbidity from a particular disease or disease in general, or its impact in terms of unfavourable consequences, or the cost of treating the victims. The burden of disease does not measure the probable success of treatment options, or the opportunity cost of measures that might be taken to reduce it.

Business case an evaluative study done from the financial perspective (q.v.) of a business.

Capabilities basic capabilities have been suggested as a useful focus for thinking about equity (q.v.). They include a person being able to do basic things, like being mobile, meet their nutritional needs, having access to clothing and shelter, the power to participate in social life.

Capacity to benefit the potential improvement in health an individual or group might achieve through improved safety measures at work, the use of health services, etc. There can be a positive capacity to benefit even when health status is falling over time, provided that the intervention in question causes it to fall less than it otherwise would.

Case-control study a study comparing individuals showing an outcome of interest, with suitable controls (q.v.) not showing that outcome.

Ceteris paribus a Latin tag meaning 'other things equal' or 'other things remaining unchanged'.

Classical statistical approach the approach to statistics in which the rules of probability are stated in terms of classical axioms.

Cohort study a longitudinal study of a group of people over time, in contrast to a cross-sectional study, which studies differences between people at a point in time.

Coincident indicator a statistical measure of events that coincide in time with the events in which one has particular interest. Compare with leading indicator (q.v.) and lagging indicator (q.v.).

Comparator an alternative technology or intervention, which may be the one in current use, employed in determining whether another technology is more or less cost-effective. Some studies may employ more than one comparator.

Compensating wage differential the idea that wage differentials compensate (or, sometimes, ought to compensate) for differences in the character of the work undertaken, like differential exposure to hazards. Taken to an extreme, it is held that wage differentials exactly compensate and so, provided one can isolate the compensation required for risk exposure from the other elements requiring compensation, one can use them to calculate the alleged value (to workers) of avoiding OHS risks.

Compensatory treatment a bias in studies that may occur in the control (q.v.) group if the intervention appears desirable, leading those assigned to control conditions to balk at their assignment, or to seek some kind of co-intervention.

Complexity theory a theory that complex social and other systems are often best studied as a whole. The idea of a complex system is that it is a functional entity, consisting not only of interdependent but also variable parts without fixed interrelationships.

Confounding this occurs when the effect of an intervention is attributed to an independent variable (q.v.) when, in fact, it is due to a different, but omitted variable (the confounder) which is correlated both with the independent and the dependent variable (q.v.) of interest.

Consensus panels meetings of experts to seek a professional agreement. Various more or less rigorous methods are used for eliciting and synthesizing opinions.

Consequence a term used in economic evaluation to describe the necessary (or predicted) future effects of a decision. In principle it embraces all the effects that may be deemed relevant, some being in monetary (for example, consequences for productivity) and others often in non-monetary forms (for example, health).

Consistency is used in a variety of senses by economists. One common meaning is that people's preferences are assumed to change little and are in this sense consistent from one period to another.

Constant prices data 'at constant prices' are those involving comparisons at different points of time from which the effects of inflation have been removed.

Constrained optimization maximizing some desired outcome subject to a resource constraint.

Consultative process a process that entails decision makers consulting people to gain access to the expertise and opinions of those with an interest in the outcome of a decision.

Contingent valuation same as stated preference (q.v.).

Contingent work work with one or more of the following characteristics: it is temporary, lacking in job security, part time, and paid on a piece work basis. Sometimes low wages are also implied, since there are many highly paid piece rate workers (for example, in film and theatre, where there are, however, also many low-paid workers). The term generally has negative connotations.

Control in longitudinal studies this is an individual without the disease or exposure being investigated or one not receiving the intervention whose effects are being investigated. In case-control studies it is an individual not exhibiting the outcome of interest.

Cost shifting a process, often though not necessarily, market driven, through which the initial incidence (q.v.) of costs is shifted from one person, organization or group to another. A common form is when rising costs, additional taxes, or premiums on firms are passed on (at least in part) to consumers in the form of higher prices.

Cost–benefit analysis a method of comparing the costs and the (money-valued) benefits of alternative interventions over a period of time. It usually requires the calculation of present values (q.v.) using a discount rate (q.v.).

Cost–consequences analysis a method of comparing technologies (q.v.) similar to cost–benefit analysis (q.v.), and cost-effectiveness analysis (q.v.), but using disaggregated costs and consequences of options without attempting to add or combine them in any way or to assign monetary or other values to all of them.

Cost-effectiveness acceptability curve (CEAC) a graphical way of showing more information about uncertainty in a cost-effectiveness analysis than can be done by using only confidence intervals. The CEAC shows the proportion of estimates of the incremental cost-effectiveness ratios (q.v.) that are lower than a variety of possible incremental cost-effectiveness ceiling ratios or thresholds.

Cost-effectiveness analysis a method of comparing the costs and the effects of alternative interventions over a period of time. It usually requires the calculation of present values (q.v.) using a discount rate (q.v.). The health outcomes, in contrast to cost–benefit analysis (q.v.), are usually left in natural units like 'reduced days of incapacity', rather than being in money terms. An intervention is usually evaluated through a comparison with some alternative, such as the status quo or a rival intervention. Not all analysts differentiate between this and cost–utility analysis (q.v.).

Cost-effectiveness ratio the ratio of cost to the output or outcome in a cost-effectiveness analysis (q.v.); or the ratio of the cost difference between two technologies and their outcome difference.

Cost-effectiveness the effect on health and other outcomes of an intervention subject to a limit on the available resources for its implementation or, equivalently, the resource cost necessary to achieve a given effect on health and other outcomes, usually relative to some alternative such as the status quo or a rival intervention.

Cost-efficiency analysis same as cost-effectiveness analysis (q.v.).

Cost-minimization analysis a simplified form of cost-effectiveness analysis (q.v.) in which cost is the dominant determining factor in a choice between alternatives, with the outcome or the value of the outcome being for practical purposes the same for each alternative.

Cost–utility analysis a method of comparing the costs and the effects of alternative interventions over a period of time. It usually requires the calculation of present values (q.v.) using a discount rate (q.v.). The health outcomes, in contrast to cost–benefit (q.v.) or cost-effectiveness (q.v.) analysis, are usually in artificial units like Quality-Adjusted Life-Years (q.v.).

Cost–utility ratio same as cost-effectiveness ratio (q.v.) save that the measure of effect is in constructed, rather than natural units.

Data dearth an absence of relevant data of suitable quality for analytical purposes.

Decision analysis a quantitative way of making decisions under conditions of uncertainty in which probabilities are attached to costs and quantities.

Decision rule a criterion (or set of criteria) to aid a decision maker in selecting between alternative courses of action. In cost-effectiveness (q.v.) contexts the rule might be 'adopt all projects for which the incremental cost-effectiveness ratio (q.v.) exceeds a given threshold'.

Deliberative process a process that not only involves consultation (q.v.), but also engages interested stakeholders in the decision-making process itself. It is characterized by the careful, deliberate consideration, and discussion of the advantages and disadvantages of various options in an effort to assist people in making a decision.

Dependent variable a variable that is postulated to be determined by one or more independent variables (q.v.).

Depreciation the change in the value of a capital good over time, usually expressed annually. The value will typically fall due to wear and tear, supercession by other capital items, or through changes in fashion. When the value rises, the term is 'appreciation'. The values in question are in constant prices: allowance having been made for inflation (q.v.).

Desert the extent to which someone deserves to receive health care, be protected from workplace accidents, etc.

Deterministic sensitivity analysis sensitivity analyses in which point estimates, rather than distributions of parameters, are varied.

Direct cost the internal cost of an activity or decision in terms of the resources used by the agency making the decision in question. It includes the cost of labour, other goods and services, capital (usually considered as a rental value) and consumables. It excludes external costs and indirect costs (q.v.). It also usually excludes any proportion of a cost that is not embodied in the price.

Disability-Adjusted Life-Year often abbreviated to DALY, this is a measure of the burden of disability-causing disease and injury. Age-specific expected life-years are adjusted for expected loss of healthy life during those years, yielding states of health measures. When two streams of DALYs are compared, potential health gain or loss is identified as between different scenarios, or as a consequence of different decisions.

Disability the so-called 'medical model' definition usually runs thus: a physical or mental impairment (q.v.) that has a substantial and long-term adverse effect on a person's ability to carry out normal activities of daily living. The so-called 'social model' emphasizes the way in which the social and physical environment can work to people's disadvantage. Legal definitions also abound and are critically important in terms of people's entitlements to various benefits.

Discount rate the rate of interest used when discounting (q.v.) to calculate a present value (q.v.).

Discounting a procedure for reducing costs or benefits occurring at different times to a common point in time, usually the present, by use of an appropriate discount rate (q.v.).

Distributive justice same as equity (q.v.) in the distribution of something.

Dominance 'strong dominance' is when one intervention is both more effective and less costly than an alternative. 'Weak dominance' is when effectiveness is higher for one intervention than another but costs are the same; or when costs are lower, but effectiveness is the same. 'Extended dominance' is when there is an intervention that is a linear combination of two other interventions that dominates other interventions.

Double counting the hazard of inadvertently counting the same thing twice. There are three common forms: simple errors due to incorrect arithmetic, suspicious circumstances due to fraudulent accounting practices, and subtler forms due to inadequate conceptual clarity, poor administrative records or poor accounting of resource costs.

Effect in the broadest sense, the effect of an intervention is usually taken to include all the expected outcomes (q.v.) in terms of health and other consequences (q.v.), but not the costs, whether direct or indirect (q.v.).

Effectiveness the extent to which an intervention has the desired outcome under normal circumstances that may be less than ideal.

Efficacy the extent to which an intervention has the desired outcome under ideal circumstances, as in a randomized controlled trial when full adherence is ensured.

Elasticity the responsiveness of a dependent variable (for example, output or demand) to changes in one of the variables determining it (for example, an input, price, or income), other things remaining the same. It may range between positive and negative infinity.

Embodied equity factors regarding equity (q.v.) that are embodied in the constructs used to assess efficiency (q.v.) or equity. For example, differential weights might be attached to quality-adjusted life-years (q.v.) according to a concept of fairness and, if so, equity (or at least some aspect of it) has been embodied.

Endogeneity a variable is endogenous if it is a function of other parameters or variables in the model.

Equity one of the two broad criteria commonly used to evaluate health and other public services, the other being efficiency (q.v.). Broadly similar to fairness, equity relates in general to ethical judgments about the fairness of distributions of income, wealth, health, cost, and benefit, to accessibility of health services, exposure to health-threatening hazards and so on. Although not the same as equality, equity often involves the equality of something (such as opportunity, health, accessibility), although there can also be equitable inequality. 'Horizontal equity' (q.v.) and 'vertical equity' (q.v.) are commonly distinguished. 'Procedural equity' relates to the fairness of the procedures under which decisions are reached.

Ergonomics the study of the interaction between people, their workplace and working environment, including the assessment of the physiological effects on workers of the design of tools, equipment and working methods.

Evidence-based decision making decisions based on the empirical evidence on a subject. The evidence in question is usually assumed to be scientific, rather than merely experiential or an expression of professional opinion.

Evidence-informed decision making similar to evidence-based decision making (q.v.), but with recognition that decisions normally need to be based on more than just the evidence about something, especially in the common situation, where the scientific evidence is absent, incomplete, of poor quality, or contested, and where other contentious issues may be at stake.

Exogeneity a variable is exogenous if it is not a function of other parameters (q.v.) or variables in the model.

Expected utility a utility (q.v.) number weighted by the probability of its occurrence.

Experience rating the practice in the insurance industry of determining premiums according to an insured person's or a firm's previous record of claims.

Expressed preference evidence about preferences gathered by experimental means using scales, rather than being inferred from behaviour. Same as stated preference (q.v.) and contingent valuation (q.v.).

External validity the legitimacy with which an intervention's observed effects can be generalized from the study subjects to a target population undergoing the intervention under normal circumstances.

Externality the consequences of an action by one individual or group as they fall on others. There may be external costs and external benefits. Some are pecuniary, affecting only the value of other resources (as when a new innovation makes a previously valuable resource obsolete); some are technological, affecting physically other people (communicable disease is a classic example of this type of negative externality); some are utility (q.v.) effects that impinge on the subjective values of others (as when, for example, one person feels sympathy and distress at the sickness of another, or relief at his/her recovery). This latter is sometimes known as a 'caring externality'.

Extra-welfarism a way of doing normative (q.v.) economics that admits aspects of life that are not mere preferences or utilities (q.v.). In health economics it is particularly associated with the idea that health is the maximand (q.v.), rather than utility or social welfare (q.v.). The concept of health may or may not be based on the preferences of the target population.

Fair innings the idea that elderly people have already had a fair innings (inning) in terms of their length of life so health improvements should receive a lower weight than health improvements for younger people. From cricket (baseball).

Final outcome an effect of an OHS intervention that is its final and ultimate desired outcome, preferably although not always easily measurable. It contrasts with intermediate outcomes (q.v.). For example, the final desired outcome of a planned new management system for OHS might be better health for workers, an intermediate outcome might be an improvement of the safety culture. If leading indicators (q.v.) such as these correlate with the final outcome, they may be used as surrogates.

Focus group a small group (usually 5–12) of relevant individuals meeting face to face to discuss a limited range of topics usually under the guidance of a moderator or facilitator.

Friction cost the idea that change itself is costly due to frictions in the marketplace. In the context of OHS, it usually refers to the cost in terms of lost productivity when workers are absent. Firms will usually restore initial production levels after some period of adaptation, the length of which may depend on the availability of suitable kinds of labour and on current unemployment levels.

Frictional unemployment temporary unemployment for new entrants to the labour market or for people between jobs and searching for new ones. Sometimes called 'search unemployment.' It arises because the process of matching heterogeneous jobs to heterogeneous worker preferences takes time and is itself costly.

Gross domestic product the total expenditure by residents and foreigners on domestically produced goods and services in a year. Usually referred to as GDP.

Handicap the prejudicial effect for an individual from a disability (q.v.) or impairment (q.v.), which precludes an individual from being normal or behaving normally.

Hawthorne effect an effect occurring amongst research subjects simply due to the fact of being observed by researchers. This confounding (q.v.) effect was first noticed in the Hawthorne plant of Western Electric in Cicero, Illinois, where production increased not as a consequence of actual changes in working conditions, but because there was a Harvard research team taking an active interest in working conditions in the plant and management was also taking an interest. A type of confounding factor in experiments and trials that may lead to bias. Also known as 'attention bias.'

Health promotion this usually refers to community-based programme to improve health and prevent disease, usually with a strong emphasis on the provision of information about the impact of a wide range of determinants on health, and often with the ideological aim of empowering ordinary people to make better decisions about their own and their families' health.

Health technology assessment the application of methods of economic evaluation, epidemiology, and decision theory to support evidence-informed decision making. Often referred by its abbreviation, HTA.

Health-related quality of life a class of measures of states of health or changes in such states used to measure the effectiveness of health care programmes. The Quality-Adjusted Life-Year (q.v.) is such a measure.

Horizontal equity equity (q.v.) in the treatment of apparent equals (such as persons exposed to the same occupational risk). A distribution of something (such as health, income, or health insurance costs) is said to be horizontally equitable when people who are the same in some relevant respect are treated the same. Thus, if the 'relevant respect' is need (a value judgment), then an equitable distribution is one that treats people with the same need in the same way. Characteristics such as race or sexual orientation are generally regarded as (ethically) irrelevant respects.

Human capital in its most general sense, this refers to the present value (q.v.) of the flow over time of human services, whether marketed or unmarketed. In a narrower sense, it refers to a method for evaluating the benefits of an OHS programme solely in terms of the present value of the future production that it enables.

Impairment according to the so-called 'medical model', it is damage or a weakening of physiological, psychological, or anatomical function or structure.

Incidence this has two forms: initial or formal incidence (often just called 'incidence') and final incidence. Formal incidence relates to the initial and short-term distribution of the monetary costs or benefits of an intervention across the various workplace parties: firms (owners), managers, workers, and consumers. Final incidence (sometimes called 'final burden') measures the longer-term consequences of the intervention for profits, rents, salaries, wages, and prices after all the economic adjustments to the intervention in all affected markets have taken place.

Incremental benefit the additional benefit to be had from increasing the rate of an activity or doing something different.

Incremental consequence the additional consequences (q.v.) to be had when a new intervention is introduced.

Incremental cost the additional cost to be had from increasing the rate of an activity or doing something different.

Incremental cost-effectiveness ratio the ratio of the difference between the costs of two alternatives and the difference between their effectiveness (or their outcomes).

Incremental net benefit the difference between the incremental benefit (q.v.) and the incremental cost (q.v.) of two possible interventions.

Independent variable a variable that affects other variables, but is not affected by them.

Indirect cost usually refers to the productivity effects that may be the consequence (q.v.) of a particular intervention. It is also sometimes used to refer to the costs of future medical care that an intervention may bring about (or avert) by virtue of increasing a person's length of life.

Inflation rising prices; generally measured as a change in an index of prices for all or most goods and services in an economy.

Intention to treat a method of analysis in clinical trials in which all patients who are randomly assigned to one of the treatments are analysed together, regardless of whether or not they actually received or completed that treatment.

Intermediate outcome an effect of an OHS intervention that is not its final desired outcome, but some measurable effect prior to this. For example, while the final desired outcome of a planned new management system for OHS might be better health for workers, an intermediate outcome might be an improvement of the safety culture. Leading indicators (q.v.), such as intermediate outcomes, may correlate with the final outcome and could thus be used as surrogates for it.

Internal validity the legitimacy with which one may infer that a given intervention did (or did not) produce the effect on the measured outcomes.

Interrupted time series a study design in which measurements are taken at multiple points in time before and after the implementation of an intervention.

Intervention group the group of people in an experiment or quasi-experiment receiving the intervention of interest whose experience will be compared with a control (q.v.) group. Also known as 'treatment' or 'experimental' arm of a trial.

Lagging indicator a statistical measure of events that occur after the events in which one has particular interest. For example, workplace injury rates are a lagging indicator of workplace interventions for primary prevention in OHS. Compare with leading indicator (q.v.) and coincident indicator (q.v.).

Latent variable a variable that is not directly observed but whose existence can be inferred by observing and measuring other variables with which it thought to be correlated. Also known as 'hidden variable' or 'hypothetical construct'.

Leading indicator a statistical measure of events that precede events in which one has particular interest. For example, the rate of implementation of action plans to improve OHS performance is a leading indicator of workplace injuries. Compare with coincident indicator (q.v.) and lagging indicator (q.v.).

Libertarianism the political philosophy whose root is the belief that each individual ought to have the maximum freedom to act and protection from the acts of others that is consistent with others having the same freedoms and protection. Strong support for exchangeable private property rights and the use of market mechanisms for resource allocation are characteristic of all libertarians.

Loss to follow-up a common cause of missing data, especially in long-term studies, through causes such as death or migration. Loss to follow-up occurs when researchers lose contact with participants in a trial.

Marginal benefit the (maximum) additional benefit to be had when the rate of an activity is increased.

Marginal cost the (minimum) additional cost entailed when the output rate is increased.

Marginal product usually of labour or per worker (can be of capital or any other factor of production). It is the (maximum) additional rate of output produced when additional labour-hours, machine-hours, etc. are used.

Marginal value the maximum value attached to a small increment of an input, a good or a service.

Market failure markets are said to fail whenever they fail to meet the standards of economists' models of the perfectly competitive market. The main sources of such failure are: asymmetry of information (q.v.), imperfect agency relationships (q.v.), consumer or producer irrationality (or inconsistency with the choice axioms of theoretical economics), incomplete markets (especially for risk-bearing), monopoly (q.v.), public goods (q.v.), and externalities (q.v.).

Market price the price of a resource in the market. This price may reflect the marginal value (q.v.) of resources embodied in the good or service if the market operates well.

Markov model a model in which the progress of a disease or disability with and without interventions is modelled in a sequence of time periods, each being associated with a particular measure of health, and each intermediate state having a probability of a subject moving from it to the next state.

Markov–Chain Monte-Carlo a method of simulating a Bayesian posterior distribution (q.v.).

Maximand the entity to be maximized.

Meta-analysis a means of quantitatively synthesizing the results of independent studies of the effects of an intervention.

Methodological uncertainty uncertainty regarding the correctness of the methodological choices one has made.

Model uncertainty uncertainty regarding the correctness of the model one is using.

Monopoly a market situation in which there is a single seller or producer.

Monte-Carlo simulation a form of simulation used in an economic evaluation, in which random numbers drawn from a given probability distribution repeatedly stand for the values of uncertain variables. Confidence limits are placed on the most likely value after a large number of such simulations.

Moral hazard this is of two main types. *Ex ante* moral hazard refers to the effect that being insured has on behaviour, taking more risks, etc., and thereby increasing the probability the event insured against will occur. *Ex post* moral hazard derives from the fact that being insured reduces the cost of a good or service to the insured and, hence, leads to an increase in demand by insured persons.

Morbidity a synonym for illness, often proxied by a patient's contact with a physician and the resultant diagnosis. Morbidity rates are calculated in a manner similar to that for mortality rates—especially cause- (or disease-) specific mortality rates.

Mortality rate the crude mortality rate is the total number of deaths per year divided by the population at mid-year × 1,000. The age-specific mortality rate is the mortality rate for a specific age group (e.g., 65 years and older). The sex-specific mortality rate is the mortality rate for males or females. The age- and sex-adjusted rates are weighted according to the proportion of each group in the population. The disease- or cause- specific mortality rate is the annual number of deaths from the particular disease divided by the mid-year population × 1,000.

Multivariate analysis an analysis in which there is more than one independent variable (q.v.) although it is sometimes used for analyses that have many dependent variables (q.v.) with 'multivariable' used in the case of multiple independent variables.

Multivariate matching a way of reducing bias in cohort studies.

Multivariate sensitivity analysis a form of sensitivity analysis (q.v.) in which more than two parameters (q.v.) are varied at a time. Also known as 'multi-way sensitivity analysis'.

Need the most frequently-met practical measures of need at the community level are morbidity (q.v.) and mortality (q.v.) data. They plainly imply a need for something, though one ought to bear in mind that it would make little sense to speak of a need for an ineffective intervention. Other concepts of need include capacity to benefit (q.v.). Need is often advocated as a criterion for adjusting the distribution of health care resources in the interests of fairness or equity (q.v.).

Neoclassical welfare economics a way of doing welfare economics (q.v.) that is particularly associated with the use of Pareto efficiency (q.v.).

Non-equivalent control group the comparison group in quasi-experimental research designs (q.v.).

Normative the adjective is usually taken to mean 'containing one or more social value judgements' and, hence, implying a norm or standard that ought to be aimed at. Welfare economics (q.v.) is entirely concerned with normative matters. 'Positive economics' attempts to exclude them altogether (though value judgments not infrequently lie just below the surface of alleged positive analyses).

Objective function a function (or objective) that is to be maximized (or minimized) with respect to choice variables of interest (like health) and subject to whatever constraints (like resources) may apply.

Occupational health and safety management system a system of management at the level of the organization for promoting a safe and healthy working environment.

Omitted variable bias a statistical bias that arises from not controlling for or modelling confounders in multivariate analyses.

Opportunity cost the value of a resource in its most highly valued alternative use. It is the most highly valued alternative that is necessarily forgone by using resources for something else. In markets this is signalled by its price but it is often helpful to state it in terms of a real and relevant entity, such as health. In the absence of markets (as in the case of allocation decision within an organization) judgment needs to be exercised in assessing opportunity cost.

Outcome a general term applied to the consequences (q.v.) of an intervention. It is often preferred to 'output' so as to avoid the impression that only goods and services constitute desired consequences. The treatment of cost-reducing effects varies. These are never counted as outputs, sometimes counted as outcomes, sometimes counted as neither, and are deducted from costs. The most common sense of outcome in health economics is 'change in health status' (which may be positive, negative or zero).

Output similar to 'outcome' (q.v.).

Parameter uncertainty uncertainty regarding the correct values of parameters.

Parameter often loosely used to refer to any factor that determines a range of variations or one that restricts the number or types of outcomes of a process. More technically, in economics and epidemiology, it refers to a constant in an equation.

Pareto efficiency an allocation of resources is considered Pareto efficient if there is no way to reallocate them (with compensation to losers) such that one or more individuals can be made better off without making someone else worse off in terms of their net utility (q.v.). This is a restrictive concept of efficiency, since it limits the types of change that can be made to ones that are voluntary and fully compensated. Similar to allocative efficiency (q.v.).

Participatory ergonomics the involvement of workplace parties in ergonomic (q.v.) interventions.

Perspective the viewpoint adopted for the purposes of an economic evaluation or similar study. It defines the scope and character of the costs and benefits to be examined, as well as other critical features, such as the rate of discount (q.v.). The perspective may be set by a client or determined by the analyst. Most textbooks advocate the use of the social (or societal) perspective, according to which all potential costs and benefits are included regardless of who bears or receives them. Sometimes called 'analytic perspective'.

Potential Pareto improvement this increase in social welfare (q.v.) is measured by a compensation test like 'could the gainers in principle compensate the losers and still retain a net gain?' It is a less stringent criterion than Pareto efficiency (q.v.) since it allows net utility losses and gains.

Predictive uncertainty variability associated with outcomes for homogeneous individuals.

Present value the value (usually monetary) of a stream of future benefits less costs derived by discounting (q.v.) at a suitable rate of interest.

Presenteeism being on the job but not fully functioning due to some health related limitation. For example, a worker who suffers from depression may be less able to work effectively.

Prevention commonly three kinds—primary prevention (activities designed to reduce the occurrence of new cases of injury and illness); secondary prevention (activities targeted at reducing the duration of existing injuries); tertiary prevention (activities designed to reduce the impact of established injuries and illnesses on social roles such as work).

Price index this measures the average price of a basket of goods and services, and is used to adjust prices in periods other than the base period so as to make comparisons at constant prices (q.v.). The most common is a consumer price index.

Primary prevention activities designed to reduce the occurrence of new cases of injury and illness, such as the purchase of safer equipment to reduce risk exposures. Compare with secondary (q.v.) and tertiary (q.v.) prevention.

Principal the person for whom an agent (q.v.) acts. Classically a patient, the doctor being the agent.

Probabilistic sensitivity analysis probabilistic sensitivity analysis attempts to quantify the uncertainty in an economic evaluation by using probability distributions over parameter values, rather than point estimates.

Procedural equity the fairness or equity (q.v.) and transparency of the procedures under which decisions are reached.

Productivity cost a substitute term for indirect cost (q.v.) or for a part of indirect costs. It is often chosen so as to avoid confusion with the accountants' usage of 'indirect cost'. A productivity cost is the opportunity cost (q.v.) of an individual's time not spent in productive work activity and it is generally conceived as including valued uses for leisure time.

Proxy an agent, substitute person, or measure acting on behalf of (or taking the place of) another; an act (such as a vote cast) so performed.

Public good in economics a public good is one that it is not possible to exclude people from consuming once any is produced (defence is a classic example). Public goods are non-rival in the sense that providing more for one person does not entail others having any less. It is not part of the definition of a public good that it be produced publicly, rather than privately, nor is it part of the definition that it be provided free of charge.

Purchasing power the command over goods and services represented by a given sum of money.

Quality-Adjusted Life-Year a measure of health which incorporates the effects of interventions both on mortality, through changes in survival duration, and morbidity, through effects on health-related quality of life (q.v.). Usually abbreviated to QALY. When two streams of QALYs are compared, potential health gain or loss is identified as between different scenarios, or as a consequence of different decisions.

Quasi-experimental study design a research design in which the assignment of subjects to comparator groups is not random or in which a control (q.v.) group is not used. Compare with randomized controlled trial (q.v.).

Randomization allocating subjects to alternative interventions or controls in a research study by chance.

Randomized controlled trial a clinical trial in which patients are allocated to treatments (including placebo) in a random fashion. The essential idea is that randomization removes confounding effects and reduces bias in the result. Also known as a randomized clinical trial. The abbreviation 'RCT' is frequently met.

Rate group a rate group consists of all employers in a workers' compensation system (q.v.) grouped by the type of business they operate (farming, forestry, nursing homes, etc.) because they have similar intrinsic health risk exposures.

Rationality economists use this term to describe behaviour that is consistent with the axioms of utility (q.v.) or expected utility theory.

Rawlsian maximin the idea that social and economic arrangements ought to be so ordered that any inequality serves the interests of those who are least well off. Also known as the 'difference principle.'

Recall bias a bias (q.v.) in data that arises from people's imperfect memories of events they are being asked to remember.

Reference case a stipulation of the features required for an evaluative study design to be regarded as scientifically satisfactory. Its purpose in health economics is also to provide consistency in the methods used, regardless of the disease areas or interventions being evaluated.

Regression to the mean an empirical phenomenon in which extreme values tend to be followed by more normal ones. For example, parents of exceptional longevity tend to have less long-lived children.

Replacement cost approach a method of estimating the value of non-paid work (e.g., of housewives) by valuing the work at the price of the paid labour that would be required to replace the unpaid.

Return on investment strictly, the discount rate (q.v.) that makes the present value (q.v.) of a future stream of monetized costs and benefits from an investment equal to zero.

Revealed preference willingness to pay (q.v.) for something as revealed by, for example, market transactions or controlled experiments. The emphasis is on the preference being revealed through behaviour in the form of a real act of choice or a hypothetical one, rather than through mere introspection.

Rule of rescue the rule of rescue is sometimes suggested as a consideration to be brought to bear in a decision normally based on the cost-effectiveness of an intervention when the incremental cost-effectiveness ratio (q.v.) is highly unfavourable and it is thought it should be overruled—such as when there is only one treatment option, death is imminent, and the situation occurs rarely.

Second best a theorem in welfare economics (q.v.) to the effect that correcting one or more, but not all, market failures (q.v.) will not necessarily increase social welfare (q.v.). The basic idea is that by correcting one imperfection you might exacerbate the bad consequences of another one.

Choosing the second best when the first best seems out of reach is thus not simply a matter of putting right each imperfection, one by one.

Secondary prevention activities targeted at reducing the duration of existing injuries and illnesses through, for example, early reporting and treatment. Compare with primary (q.v.) and tertiary (q.v.) prevention.

Selection bias one of many kinds of bias to which clinical and other trials are vulnerable. In this case, the bias arises in a sample that differs systematically in its characteristics from the general population due to a feature of the selection process. Such a bias will enter, for example, if the selection rule is 'take those whose names start with A', or 'those who work on the top floor', or 'those who respond to a mailed questionnaire'. Also refers to bias arising from pre-existing difference in comparator groups (e.g., differing age distributions).

Sensitivity analysis a procedure by which the outcomes of an evaluative analysis are tested for their responsiveness to changes in some or all of the assumptions made, or to empirical estimates that are on either side of the mid-point estimates. The object is to see whether the conclusion changes when such changes are made.

Shadow price the price of a resource or consumption good adjusted to reflect what is believed to be its true opportunity cost (q.v.) or the amount of money a consumer is willing to pay for additional units of a good or service.

Social welfare the normative (q.v.) state of a society in terms of the utilities (q.v.) or other components of wellbeing of all the members of that society.

Stated preference the preference to pay for a non-marketed entity like health as derived from questionnaires or experiments. It is stated verbally (i.e., orally or in writing), rather than revealed by actual behaviour in experiments or in real life. Another term for it is 'contingent valuation'.

Statistical power intervention trials ought to be big enough to have a high chance of detecting a statistically significant effect, and one that is also clinically or biologically significant, if one exists. More formally, power is the probability that the null hypothesis will be rejected if it is, indeed, false.

Status quo a Latin tag meaning the current state of things; the existing situation; the ways we do things now.

Study design the design of empirical studies typically falls into two broad categories—analytical and descriptive. Analytical studies are also two-fold: experimental, such as the randomized controlled trial (q.v.) and quasi-experimental, such as cohort studies (q.v.). Social surveys typify the descriptive study design.

Study group contamination a source of bias in a study in which one or more subjects (e.g., workers or managers) influence the behaviour and outcomes of others at the same site who are members of the control group.

Summary measures indicators of various kinds that combine many factors. For example, a cost-effectiveness ratio (q.v.) typically combines many costs and many outcome attributes, and is a summary measure of the cost-effectiveness (q.v.) of an intervention.

Supplier-induced demand the effect that doctors (or other professionals), as providers of services, may have in creating more patient demand than there would be if they acted as perfect agents (q.v.) for their patients. Frequently referred to by its acronym, SID.

Sustainability usually refers to the persistence with which a situation (such as the effects of an intervention) can be maintained. The long-term feasibility of ongoing effectiveness of an intervention.

Systematic review a form of literature review that seeks to minimize bias by being very explicit in its selection and evaluative procedures. Usual attributes include: explicit identification and scoping of research questions, use of explicit methods for searching the literature, explicit criteria for including or excluding material, explicit criteria for appraising quality and reliability and a systematic analysis/synthesis of research findings.

Taylor series expansion a way of approximating a function near a particular point.

Technology a term that can be used either narrowly (as in 'pharmaceutical') or broadly (as in 'workplace intervention') to describe a way of doing something, a means of accomplishing something. In health economics it was initially used to describe tools such as scanners, prescription drugs, bed rest, and watchful waiting. It is increasingly applied also to the evaluation of methods of governance and management.

Tertiary prevention activities designed to reduce the impact of established injuries and illnesses on social roles, such as work, by restoring functional ability or role performance through accommodation and vocational rehabilitation. Compare with primary (q.v.) and secondary (q.v.) prevention.

Testing effect an artefact created by pre-intervention measurement.

Theory of change comprises a model of how change is predicted to take place in an organization following some intervention. The model typically specifies its assumptions, the decision-making processes, and short-, medium-, and long-term consequences.

Third party payer an insurance agency or similar agency responsible for paying for, rather than directly providing, health care.

Time frame either the period of time over which observations have been made in a study or the definition of 'period' when rates of something are being measured (e.g., so much per week, per month).

Time preference the phenomenon that future benefits are less preferred by an individual than those closer in date, and more distant costs are regarded as less burdensome than those in immediate prospect.

Transfer payment a transfer of purchasing power from one individual or group to another that is not a compensation for parting with the ownership of something (like a consumable item or labour). It is usually made for the purpose of social equity (q.v.) or, as is the case with subsidies, to provide incentives for people to behave in particular ways.

Transfer price an administrative price at which one department or other section of a firm sells its products to other parts of the same firm.

Uncertainty two kinds are commonly considered: stochastic uncertainty (sometimes called 'first-order uncertainty') and subjective uncertainty (sometimes called 'second-order uncertainty'). The first is uncertainty arising from randomness in the data being studied, the second arises from insufficient knowledge about the parameters (q.v.) of the analysis.

Univariate sensitivity analysis a form of sensitivity analysis (q.v.) in which one parameter (q.v.) is varied at a time.

Utility an abstract way of ordering a person's preferences by assigning numbers to bundles of goods and services, or to characteristics of goods or services. Higher numbers indicate greater utility or satisfaction. Utility can be measured ordinally, indicating no more than the ranking, or cardinally on linear scale in the way temperature is measured, or (again cardinally, but more strongly) on a ratio scale in the way that distance and weight are measured.

Value-of-information an approach to uncertainty in an economic evaluation emphasizing that the main reason for examining the uncertainty surrounding outcomes of interest is to ascertain the value of acquiring additional information, for example, through research, in order to reduce future uncertainty and so inform future related decisions better.

Vertical equity equity (q.v.) in the treatment of apparent unequals (such as persons with different occupational health exposures). A distribution is said to be vertically equitable when people who are different in some relevant respect are treated appropriately differently. Thus, if the relevant respect is need, an equitable distribution will accord more (of some relevant entity) to those in greater need of it. If the relevant respect is ability to pay, an equitable distribution of the burden of funding entails the richer paying more (perhaps proportionately more or, as in progressive tax structures, more than proportionately more) than others. How much more is equitable will of course entail further value judgments.

Welfare economics the branch of economics concerned with identifying the conditions that make for a good society, and identifying changes in allocations of goods and services, or arrangements for allocating goods and services, which are better for society.

Welfarism the idea that human welfare can be adequately addressed in terms of the satisfaction of individual preferences (utilities) and nothing much more.

Willingness to accept the minimum someone requires in order to voluntarily relinquish a good or service.

Willingness to pay the maximum someone will pay to acquire a good or service.

Within-individual variability the sort of variability in outcome that results even when individuals are homogeneous (q.v.).

Work role functioning a measure of a worker's ability to do the job. Simple categorizations may be used, such as 'not working', 'working with limitations', 'working well'.

Workers' compensation insurance programmes through which workers may receive compensation in the event of an occupational injury or disease. The role sometimes includes payment for health care needed following such events or even the direct provision of some health care services. Funding usually comes from premiums paid by employers.

Bibliography

Acton JP (1976). *Evaluating public programs to save lives: the case of heart attacks.* RAND Corporation, Santa Monica, Report No. R950RC.

Adelman JU, Sharfman M, Johnson R, *et al.* (1996). Impact of oral sumatriptan on workplace productivity, health-related quality of life, health care use, and patient satisfaction with medication in nurses with migraine. *American Journal of Managed Care*, **10**, 1407–16.

Ades AE, Lu G, and Claxton K (2003). Expected value of sample information calculations in medical decision modelling. *Medical Decision Making*, **243**, 207–27.

Alchian AA (1959). Costs and outputs. In M Abramovitz (ed) *The allocation of economic resources*, pp. 23–45. Stanford University Press, Stanford.

Alchian AA (1965). Some economics of property rights. *Il Politico*, **30**, 816–29.

Alchian AA (1968). Cost. In DL Sills and RK Merton (eds) *International encyclopedia of the social sciences: Volume 3.* Crowell, Collier & Mcmillan, New York, pp. 404–15.

Amick III BC and Gimeno D (2007). Measuring work outcomes with a focus on health-related productivity loss. In D Carr and H Wittink (eds) *Pain management: evidence, outcomes, and quality of life, a sourcebook.* Elsevier, Edinburgh, pp. 329–43.

Amick III BC, Robertson MM, DeRango K, Bazzani L, Moore A, Rooney T, and Harrist R (2003). Effects of an office ergonomic intervention on musculoskeletal symptoms. *Spine*, **28**, 2706–11.

Amick III BC, Habeck RV, Ossmann J, Fossel AH, Keller R, and Katz JN (2004). Predictors of successful work role functioning after carpal tunnel release surgery. *Journal of Occupational and Environmental Medicine*, **46**, 490–500.

Andrews DWK (1993). Tests for parameter instability and structural change with unknown change point. *Econometrica*, **61**, 821–56.

Arnesen T and Trommald M (2004). Roughly right or precisely wrong? Systematic review of quality-of-life weights elicited with the time trade-off method. *Journal of Health Services Research Policy*, **9**, 43–50.

Arnetz BB, Sjögren B, Rydéhn B, and Meisel R (2003). Early workplace intervention for employees with musculoskeletal-related absenteeism: a prospective controlled intervention study. *Journal of Occupational and Environmental Medicine*, **45**, 499–506.

Baxter K and Harrison D (2000). A simple cost benefit analysis for an ergonomics 'train-the-trainer' program. In *Ergonomics for the new millennium.* Human Factors and Ergonomics Society, San Diego, California, USA, pp. 1–3.

Beatson M and Coleman M (1997). International comparisons of the economic costs of work accidents and work-related ill health. In J Mossink and F Licher (eds) *Costs and benefits of occupational safety and health: proceedings of the European Conference on Costs and Benefits of Occupational Safety and Health.* NIA TNO B.V., Amsterdam.

Beattie J, Chilton S, Cookson R, *et al.* (1998a). *Valuing health and safety controls: a literature review.* HSE Books, London, Contract Research Report 171/1998.

Beattie J, Covey J, Dolan P, *et al.* (1998b). On the contingent valuation of safety and the safety of contingent valuation: part 1—caveat investigator. *Journal of Risk and Uncertainty*, **17**, 5–25.

Belkic KL, Schwartz J, and Schnall PL (2000). Evidence for mediating econeurocardiologic mechanisms. In PL Schnall, KL Belkic, P Landisbergis, and D Maker (eds) *The workplace and cardiovascular disease. occupational medicine: state of the art reviews in occupational medicine.* Hanley & Belfus, Philadelphia.

Belkic KL, Landsbergis PA, Schnall PL, and Baker D (2004). Is job strain a major source of cardiovascular disease risk? *Scandinavian Journal of Work, Environment & Health*, **30**, 85–128.

Berndt ER, Bailit HL, Keller MB, Verner JC, and Finkelstein SN (2000). Health care use and at-work productivity among employees with mental disorders. *Health Affairs*, **19**, 244–56.

Betcherman G (1995). Inside the black box: human resource management and the labor market. In RJ Adams, G Betcherman, and B Bilson (eds) *Good jobs, bad jobs, no jobs: tough choices for Canadian Labor Law.* CD Howe Institute, Toronto, pp. 70–97.

Birch S and Gafni A (1992). Cost-effectiveness/utility analyses: do current decision rules lead us to where we want to be? *Journal of Health Economics*, **11**, 279–96.

Blades CA, Culyer AJ, and Walker A (1987). Health service efficiency: appraising the appraisers—a critical review of economic appraisal in practice. *Social Science & Medicine*, **25**, 461–72.

Blane D, Power C, and Bartley M (1996). Illness behaviour and the measurement of class differentials in morbidity. *Journal of the Royal Statistical Society Association*, **59**, 77–92.

Blomquist GC (2004). Self-protection and averting behavior, values of statistical lives, and benefit cost analysis of environmental policy. *Review of Economics of the Household*, **2**, 89–110.

Boden LJ and Galizzi M (1999). Economic consequences of workplace injuries and illnesses: Lost earnings and benefit adequacy. *American Journal of Industrial Medicine*, **36**, 487–503.

Bond TJ, Galinsky E, and Swanberg JE (1998). *The 1997 national study of the changing workforce.* Families and Work Institute, New York.

Borg W, Kristensen TS, and Burr H (2000). Work environment and changes in self-rated health: a five year follow-up study. *Stress Medicine*, **16**, 37–47.

Bosma H, Marmot MG, Hemingway H, Nicholson A, Brunner E, and Stansfeld S (1997). Low job control and risk of coronary heart disease in Whitehall II (prospective cohort) study. *British Medical Journal*, **314**, 558–65.

Bosma H, Peter R, Siegrist J, and Marmot M (1998). Two alternative job stress models and the risk of coronary heart disease. *American Journal of Public Health*, **88**, 68–74.

Bradley W (1996). Management and prevention of on the job injuries. *AAOHN Journal*, **44**, 402–5.

Briggs AH (2000). Handling uncertainty in cost-effectiveness models. *Pharmacoeconomics*, **17**, 479–500.

Briggs AH and Fenn P (1998). Confidence intervals or surfaces? Uncertainty on the cost-effectiveness plane. *Health Economics*, **7**, 723–40.

Briggs AH, Sculpher M, and Buxton M (1994). Uncertainty in the economic evaluation of health care technologies: the role of sensitivity analysis. *Health Economics*, **3**, 95–104.

Brouwer WBF, Koopmanschap MA, and Rutten FF (1997). Productivity costs measurement through quality of life? A response to the recommendation of the Washington Panel. *Health Economics*, **6**, 253–9.

Brouwer WBF, van Exel NJA, Koopmanschap MA, and Rutten FF (2002). Productivity costs before and after absence from work: as important as common? *Health Policy*, **61**, 173–87.

Brunner E (1996). The social and biological basis of cardiovascular disease in office workers. In D Blane, E Brunner, and R Wilkinson (eds) *Health and social organization*. Routledge, London.

Bunn WB, Pikelny DB, Paralkar S, Slavin T, Borden S, and Allen HM (2003). The burden of allergies—and the capacity of medications to reduce this burden—in a heavy manufacturing environment. *Journal of Occupational and Environmental Medicine*, **45**, 941–55.

Burton WN, Conti DJ, Chen CY, Schultz AB, and Edington DW (1999). The role of health risk factors and disease on worker productivity. *Journal of Occupational and Environmental Medicine*, **41**, 863–77.

Burton WN, Conti DJ, Chen CY, Schultz AB, and Edington DW (2001). The impact of allergies and allergy treatment on worker productivity. *Journal of Occupational and Environmental Medicine*, **43**, 64–71.

Carson RT and Mitchell RC (1995). Sequencing and nesting in contingent valuation surveys. *Journal of Environmental Economics and Management*, 28, 155–74.

Carthy T, Chilton S, Covy J, *et al.* (1999). On the contingent valuation of safety and the safety of contingent valuation: part 2—the CV/SG 'chained' approach. *Journal of Risk and Uncertainty*, **17**, 187–213.

Castells M and Aoyama Y (1994). Paths towards the informational society: employment structure in G-7 countries, 1920–90. *International Labour Review*, **133**, 6–33.

Champoux D and Brun JP (2003). Occupational health and safety management in small size enterprises: an overview of the situation and avenues for intervention and research. *Safety Science*, **41**, 301–18.

Chodick G, Lerman Y, Wood F, Aloni H, Peled T, and Ashkenazi S (2002). Cost–utility analysis of hepatitis A prevention among health care workers in Israel. *Journal of Occupational and Environmental Medicine*, **44**, 109–15.

Claxton K, Sculpher M, McCabe C, *et al.* (2005). Probabilistic sensitivity analysis for NICE technology assessment: not an optional extra. *Health Economics*, **14**, 339–47.

Cole DC, Wells RP, Frazer MB, Kerr MS, Neumann WP, and Laing AC (2003). Methodological issues in evaluating workplace interventions to reduce work-related musculoskeletal disorders through mechanical exposure reduction. *Scandinavian Journal of Work, Environment & Health*, **29**, 396–405.

Commonwealth Department of Health, Housing and Community Services (1992). Guidelines for the pharmaceutical industry on preparation of submissions to the Pharmaceutical Benefits Advisory Committee. Canberra: AGPS.

Cook TD and Campbell DT (1979). *Quasi-experimentation: design and analysis issues for field settings*. Rand McNally College Publishing, Chicago.

Cook TD, Campbell DT, and Peraccio L (1990). Quasi experimentation. In MD Dunnette and LM Hough (eds) *Handbook of industrial and organizational psychology*. Consulting Psychologists Press Inc, Palo Alto, California.

Cookson R (2000). Incorporating psycho-social considerations into health valuations: an experimental study. *Journal of Health Economics*, **19**, 369–401.

Cookson R and Dorman P (2008). *Lessons from the literature on valuing reductions in physical risk*. Institute for Work & Health Toronto, Working Paper #342.

Cookson R, McCabe C, and Tsuchiya A (2007). *Public health care resource allocation and the rule of rescue*. University of Sheffield Health Economics and Decision Science Discussion Paper 07/04.

Cooper H and Hedges LV (1994). *The handbook of research synthesis*. Russell Sage Foundation, New York.

Courtney TK and Webster BS (1999). Disabling occupational morbidity in the United States: an alternative way of seeing the Bureau of Labor Statistics' data. *Journal of Occupational and Environmental Medicine*, **41**, 60–9.

Covey J, Jones-Lee M, Loomes G, and Robinson A (1995). *The exploratory empirical study*. University of East Anglia, MAFF Report, Contract No. 1A021.

Culyer AJ (1987). The scope and limits of health economics (with reference to economic appraisals of health services). In *Oekonomie des Gesundheitswesen, Jahrestagung des Vereins für Socialpolitik, Gesellschaft für Wirtschafts- und Sozialwissenschaften, Neue Folge Band*, **159**, pp. 31–53.

Culyer AJ (1989). The normative economics of health care finance and provision. *Oxford Review of Economic Policy*, **5**, 34–58.

Culyer AJ (1991). The normative economics of health care finance and provision. In A McGuire, P Fenn, and K Mayhew (eds) *Providing health care: the economics of alternative systems of finance and delivery*. Oxford University Press, Oxford, pp. 65–98.

Culyer AJ (2006). The bogus conflict between efficiency and equity. *Health Economics*, **15**, 1155–8.

Culyer AJ (2007). Need: an instrumental view. In R Ashcroft, A Dawson, H Draper, and J McMillan (eds) *Principles of health core ethics*. Wiley, Chichester, pp. 231–38.

Culyer AJ and Lomas J (2006). Deliberative processes and evidence-informed decision-making in health care—do they work and how might we know? *Evidence and Policy*, **2**, 357–71.

Daniels N (1985). *Just health care*. Cambridge University Press, Cambridge.

Daniels N (2000). Accountability for reasonableness. *British Medical Journal*, **321**, 1300–1.

Daniels N and Sabin JE (1998). The ethics of accountability in managed care reform. *Health Affairs*, **17**, 50–64.

Daniels PW (1993). *Service industries in the world economy*. Blackwell, Oxford.

de Blaeij A, Florax RJGM, Rietveld P, and Verhoef E (2003). The value of statistical life in road safety: a meta-analysis. *Accident Analysis and Prevention*, **35**, 973–86.

Deeks JJ, Dinnes J, D'Amico R, *et al.* (2003). Evaluating non-randomised intervention studies. *Health Technology Assessment*, **7**, 1–173.

Dehejia RH and Wahba S (1999). Causal effects in non-experimental studies: re-evaluating the evaluation of training programs. *Journal of the American Statistical Association*, **94**, 1053–62.

Department for Transport (2007). *Highway economics note number 1: 2005 valuation of the benefits of prevention of road accidents and casualties*. HMSO, London.

DeRango K and Franzini L (2003). Economic evaluations of workplace health interventions: theory and literature review. In JC Quick and LE Tetrick (eds) *Handbook of occupational health psychology*. American Psychological Association, Washington, DC, pp. 417–30.

DeRango K, Amick III BC, Robertson M, Rooney T, Moore A, and Bazzani L (2003). *The productivity consequences of two ergonomic interventions.* Institute for Work & Health, Toronto, Working Paper #222.

Dolan P and Olsen JA (2002). *Distributing health care: economic and ethical issues.* Oxford University Press, Oxford.

Donaldson C, Gerard K, Mitton C, Jan S, and Wiseman V (2005). *Economics of health care financing: the visible hand* (2nd edn). Palgrave Macmillan, Houndmills.

Dorman P (1996). *Markets and mortality: economics, dangerous work, and the value of human life.* Cambridge University Press, New York.

Dorman P (2000). *The economics of safety, health, and well-being at work: an overview.* InFocus Program on SafeWork, International Labour Organisation, The Evergreen State College, Olympia.

Dorman P and Hagstrom P (1998). Wage compensation for dangerous work revisited. *Industrial and Labour Relations Review*, **52**, 116–33.

Draper D (1995). Assessment and propagation of model uncertainty (with discussion). *Journal of the Royal Statistical Society, Series B*, **57**, 45–97.

Driscoll T, Takala J, Steenland K, Corvalan C, and Fingerhut M (2005). Review of estimates of the global burden of injury and illness due to occupational exposures. *American Journal of Industrial Medicine*, **48**, 491–502.

Drummond M and Sculpher M (2005). Common methodological flaws in economic evaluations. *Medical Care*, **43**, 5–14.

Drummond M, Sculpher M, Torrance GW, O'Brien BJ, and Stoddart GL (2005). *Methods for the economic evaluation of health care programmes.* Oxford University Press, Oxford.

Dubourg WR, Loomes G, and Jones-Lee MW (1997). Imprecise preferences and survey design in contingent valuation. *Economica*, **64**, 681–702.

Duffy A and Pupo N (1992). *Part-time paradox: connecting gender, work and family.* McClelland & Stewart, Toronto.

Duffy A, Glenday D, and Pupo N (1997). *Good jobs, bad jobs, no jobs: the transformation of work in the 21st century.* Harcourt Brace, Toronto.

Dumaine B (1994). The trouble with teams. *Fortune*, **130**, 86–92.

Eakin JM (1992). Leaving it up to the workers: sociological perspective on the management of health and safety in small workplaces. *International Journal of Health Services*, **22**, 689–704,

Egger M, Smith GD, and Altman DG (2003). *Systematic reviews in health care: meta-analysis in context.* BMJ Books, London.

European Foundation (1997). *Time constraints and autonomy at work in the European Union.* European Foundation for the Improvement of Living and Working Conditions, Dublin.

Fahs MC, Markowitz SB, Leigh JP, Shin CG, and Landrigan PJ (1997). A national estimate of the cost of occupationally related disease in 1992. *Annals of the New York Academy of Sciences*, **837**, 440–55.

Farr W (1853). The income and property tax. *Journal of the Statistical Society of London*, **16**, 1–44.

Fenwick E, Claxton K, and Sculpher M (2001). Representing uncertainty: the role of cost-effectiveness acceptability curves. *Health Economics*, **10**, 779–87.

Fenwick E, Marshall DA, Levy AR, and Nichol G (2006). Using and interpreting cost-effectiveness acceptability curves: an example using data from a trial of management strategies for atrial fibrillation. *BMC Health Services Research*, **6**, 52.

Fisher RA (1973). *Statistical methods for research workers*. Hafner, New York.

Folland S, Goodman AC, and Stano M (2004). *The economics of health and health care* (4th edn). Pearson Prentice Hall, Upper Saddle River.

Frank J and Maetzel A (2000). Determining occupational disorder: can this camel carry more straw? In TJ Sullivan (ed) *Injury and the new world of work*. University of British Columbia Press, Vancouver.

Gafni A and Birch S (2003). Inclusion of drugs in provincial drug benefit programs: should reasonable decisions lead to uncontrolled growth in expenditures? *Canadian Medical Association Journal*, **168**, 849–51.

Gallie D (2000). The polarization of the labor market and exclusion of vulnerable groups. In K Isaksson, C Hogstedt, C Ericksson, and T Theorell (eds) *Health effects of the new labor market*. Plenum Publishers, New York.

Garber AM and Phelps CE (1997). Economic foundations of cost-effectiveness analysis. *Journal of Health Economics*, **16**, 1–31.

Gardner D, Carlopio J, Fonteyn PN, and Cross JA (1999). Mechanical equipment injuries in small manufacturing businesses. Knowledge, behavioural, and management issues. *International Journal of Occupational Safety and Ergonomics*, **5**, 59–71.

Garland MJ (1992). Rationing in public: Oregon's priority-setting methodology. In MA Strosberg, JM Wiener, RB Baker and IA Fein (eds) *Rationing America's medical care: the Oregon Plan and beyond: papers*. Brookings Institution, Washington, DC, pp. 37–59.

Gegax D, Gerking S, and Schulze W (1991). Perceived risk and the marginal value of safety. *Review of Economics and Statistics*, **73**, 589–96.

Gilkey DP, Bigelow PL, Herron RE, Greinstein S, Chadwick BR, and Fowler JK (1998). The HomeSafe Pilot Program: a novel approach to injury prevention in residential construction. *Work*, **10**, 167–80.

Gilkey DP, Hautaluoma JE, Ahmed TP, Keefe TJ, Herron RE, and Bigelow PL (2003a). Construction work practices and conditions improved after 2 years' participation in the HomeSafe pilot program. *AIHA Journal*, **64**, 346–51.

Gilkey DP, Keefe TJ, Hautaluoma JE, Bigelow PL, Herron RE, and Stanley SA (2003b). Management commitment to safety and health in residential construction: HomeSafe spending trends 1991–1999. *Work*, **20**, 35–44.

Goetzel RZ, Ozminkowski RJ, Baase CM, and Billotti GM (2005). Estimating the return-on-investment from changes in employee health risks on the Dow Chemical Company's health care costs. *Journal of Occupational and Environmental Medicine*, **47**, 759–68.

Gold MR, Siegel JE, Russell LB, and Weinstein MC (1996). *Cost-effectiveness in health and medicine*. Oxford University Press, New York.

Gold MR, Stevenson D, and Fryback DG (2002). HALYS and QALYS and DALYS, Oh My: similarities and differences in summary measures of population health. *Annual Review of Public Health*, **23**, 115–34.

Goldenhar LM and Schulte PA (1994). Intervention research in occupational health and safety. *Journal of Occupational Medicine*, **36**, 763–75.

Goldenhar LM and Schulte PA (1996). Methodological issues for intervention research in occupational health and safety. *American Journal of Industrial Medicine*, **29**, 289–94.

Goldenhar LM, Ruder AM, Ewers LM, Earnest S, Haag WM, and Petersen MR (1999). Concerns of the dry-cleaning industry: a qualitative investigation of labor and management. *American Journal of Industrial Medicine*, **35**, 112–23.

Goldenhar LM, LaMontagne AD, Katz T, Heaney C, and Landsbergis P (2001). The intervention research process in occupational safety and health: an overview from the National Occupational Research Agenda Intervention Effectiveness Research team. *Journal of Occupational and Environmental Medicine*, **43**, 616–22.

Goossens ME, Evers SM, Vlaeyen JW, Rutten-an Mölken MP, and van der Linden SMJP (1999). Principles of economic evaluation for interventions of chronic musculoskeletal pain. *European Journal of Pain*, **3**, 343–53.

Gravelle H and Smith D (2001). *Discounting for health effects in cost–benefit and cost-effectiveness analysis*. The University for York, Centre for Health Economics, York, CHE Technical Paper Series 20.

Graetz B (1993). Health consequences of employment and unemployment: longitudinal evidence for young men and women. *Social Science & Medicine*, **36**, 715–24.

Greenwood JG, Wolf HJ, Pearson JC, Woon CL, Posey P, and Main CF (1990). Early intervention in low back disability among coal miners in West Virginia: negative findings. *Journal of Occupational Medicine*, **32**, 1047–52.

Haddix AC, Teutsch SM, and Corso P (2003). *Prevention effectiveness: a guide to decision analysis and economic evaluation*. Oxford University Press, New York.

Hagard S and Carter FA (1976). Preventing the birth of infants with Down's syndrome: a cost–benefit analysis. *British Medical Journal*, **1**, 753–56.

Hajer MA and Wagenaar H (2003). *Deliberative policy analysis: understanding governance in the network society*. Cambridge University Press, Cambridge.

Hausman DM and McPherson MS (2006). *Economic analysis, moral philosophy, and public policy* (2nd edn). Cambridge University Press, Cambridge.

Health Canada (1998). *Economic burden of illness in Canada, 1998*. Health Canada, Ottawa.

Hemingway H and Marmot M (1999). Psychosocial factors in the aetiology and prognosis of coronary heart disease: systematic review of prospective cohort studies. *British Medical Journal*, **318**, 1460–7.

Hirth RA, Chernew ME, Miller E, Fendrick MF, and Weissert WG (2000). Willingness to pay for a Quality-Adjusted Life Year: in search of a standard. *Medical Decision Making*, **20**, 332–42.

Hjelmgren J, Berggren F, and Andersson F (2001). Health economic guidelines—similarities, differences and some implications. *Value Health*, **4**, 225–50.

Hobsbawm EA (1994). *Age of extremes: the short twentieth century, 1914–1991*. Abacus, London.

Hoch J and Dewa C (2007). Lessons from trial-based cost-effectiveness analyses of mental health interventions: why uncertainty about the outcome, estimate and willingness to pay matters. *Pharmacoeconomics*, **25**, 807–16.

Hoch J and Dewa C (2008). A clinician's guide to correct cost-effectiveness analysis: think incremental not average. *Canadian Journal of Psychiatry*, **53**, 267–74.

Hoch J and Smith M (2006). A guide to economic evaluation: methods for cost-effectiveness analysis of person-level data. *Journal of Traumatic Stress*, **19**, 787–97.

Hoch J, Briggs A, and Willan A (2002). Something old, something new, something borrowed, something BLUE: a framework for the marriage of health econometrics and cost-effectiveness analysis. *Health Economics*, **11**, 415–30.

Hoch J, Rockx M, and Krahn A. (2006). Using the net benefit regression framework to construct cost-effectiveness acceptability curves: an example using data from a trial of external loop recorders versus Holter monitoring for ambulatory monitoring of 'community acquired' syncope. *BMC Health Services Research*, **6**, 68.

Holmes N, Gifford TJ, Trigs SM, and Dawkins AW (1997). Occupational injury risk in a blue collar, small business industry: implications for prevention. *Safety Science*, **25**, 67–78.

Holzer HJ (1996). *What employers want: job prospects for less-educated workers*. Russell Sage Foundation, New York.

Hoover K (2000). Business groups sue to stop OSHA's ergonomic rule. *Washington Business Journal*, 17 Nov.

Howell HJ and Wolff EN (1991). Trends in the growth and distribution of skills in the U.S. workplace, 1960–1985. *Industrial and Labour Relations Review*, **44**, 486–502.

Hyatt DE and Thomason T (1998). *Evidence on the efficacy of experience rating in British Columbia*. Royal Commission on Workers' Compensation in British Columbia, Vancouver.

International Labour Organization (2003). *Safety in numbers: pointers for a global safety culture at work*. Geneva: International Labour Office.

Jensen IB, Bergström G, Ljungquist T, Bodin L, and NygrenÅL (2001). A randomized controlled component analysis of a behavioral medicine rehabilitation program for chronic spinal pain: are the effects dependent on gender? *Pain*, **91**, 65–78.

Johannesson M (1995). On the estimation of cost-effectiveness ratios. *Health Policy*, **31**, 225–9.

Johannesson M and Weinstein MC (1993). On the decision rules of cost-effectiveness analysis. *Journal of Health Economics*, **12**, 459–67.

Johns G (1994). Absenteeism estimates by employees and managers—divergent perspectives and self-serving perceptions. *Journal of Applied Psychology*, **79**, 229–39.

Jones-Lee MW (1989). *The economics of safety and physical risk*. Basil Blackwell, Oxford.

Jones-Lee MW and Loomes G (1995). Scale and context effects in the valuation of transport safety. *Journal of Risk and Uncertainty*, **11**, 183–203.

Jones-Lee MW, Hammerton M, and Phillips PR (1985). The value of safety: results of a national sample survey. *Economic Journal*, **95**, 49–92.

Jones-Lee MW, Loomes G, and Philips PR (1995). Valuing the prevention of non-fatal road injuries: contingent valuation vs standard gambles. *Oxford Economic Papers*, **47**, 676–95.

Kaplan RS and Norton DP (1992). The balanced scorecard—measures that drive performance. *Harvard Business Review*, **70**, 71–9.

Karasek R, Brisson C, Kawakami N, Houtman I, Bongers P, and Amick B (1998). The Job Content Questionnaire (JCQ): an instrument for internationally comparative assessments of psychosocial job characteristics. *Journal of Occupational Health Psychology*, **3**, 322–55.

Karlsson G and Johannesson M (1996). The decision rules of cost-effectiveness analysis. *Pharmacoeconomics*, **9**, 113–20.

Karnon J, Tsuchiya A, and Dolan P (2005). Developing a relativities approach to valuing the prevention of non-fatal work-related accidents and ill-health. *Health Economics*, **14**, 1103–15.

Kessler RC, Barber C, Beck A, *et al.* (2003). The World Health Organization Health and Work Performance Questionnaire (HPQ). *Journal of Occupational and Environmental Medicine*, **45**, 156–74.

Kessler RC, Ames M, Hymel PA, Loeppke R, McKenas DK, Richling DE, Stang PE, Ustun TB (2004). Using the World Health Organization Health and Work Performance Questionnaire (HPQ) to evaluate the indirect workplace costs of illness. *Journal of Occupational and Environmental Medicine*, **46**, S23-S37.

Kidd P, Parshall M, Wojcik S, and Struttmann T (2004). Overcoming recruitment challenges in construction safety intervention research. *American Journal of Industrial Medicine*, **45**, 297–304.

Knieser TJ and Leeth J (1991). Compensating wage differentials for fatal injury risk in Australia, Japan and the United States. *Journal of Risk and Insurance*, **4**, 75–90.

Kompier M and Cooper C (1999). *Preventing stress, improving productivity: European case studies in the workplace*. Routledge, London.

Koningsveld EA (2005). Intervention studies in occupational epidemiology. *Occupational and Environmental Medicine*, **62**, 205–10.

Koningsveld EA, Dul J, Van Rhijn GW, and Vink P (2005). Enhancing the impact of ergonomics interventions. *Ergonomics*, **48**, 559–80.

Koopmanschap MA and Rutten FFH (1996). A practical guide for calculating the indirect costs of disease. *Pharmacoeconomics*, **10**, 460–6.

Koopmanschap MA, Rutten FFH, Van Ineveld BM, and Van Roijen L (1995). The friction cost method for measuring indirect cost of disease. *Journal of Health Economics*, **14**, 171–89.

Kotter JP (1995). Leading change: why transformation efforts fail. *Harvard Business Review*, **73**, 59–67.

Krabbe PFM, Essink-Bot ML, and Bonsel GJ (1997). The comparability and reliability of five health-state valuation methods. *Social Science and Medicine*, **45**, 1641–52.

Kramer DE, Cole DC, Theberge N, and Hepburn G (2005). *Walking a mile in each others' shoes: the evolution of a research design with workplace health and safety partners as part of the process*. Institute for Work & Health, Toronto, Working Paper #309.

Kraut A (1994). Estimates of the extent of morbidity and mortality due to occupational diseases in Canada. *American Journal of Industrial Medicine*, **25**, 267–78.

Kraut A, Mustard CA, Walld R, and Tate R (2000). Unemployment and health care utilization. In K Isaksson, C Hogstedt, C Ericksson, and T Theorell (eds) *Health Effects of the New Labour Market*. Plenum Press, London.

Kristensen TS (2005). Intervention studies in occupational epidemiology. *Occupational and Environmental Medicine*, **62**, 205–10.

Kunst AE, Groenhof F, Mackenbach JP, and Health EW (1998). Occupational class and cause-specific mortality in middle aged men in eleven European countries: comparison of population based studies. *British Medical Journal*, **316**, 1636–42.

LaMontagne AD and Needleman C (1996). Overcoming practical challenges in intervention research in occupational health and safety. *American Journal of Industrial Medicine*, **29**, 367–72.

LaMontagne AD, Barbeau E, Youngstrom RA, Lewiton M, Stoddard AM, McLellan D, Wallace LM, and Sorensen G (2004). Assessing and intervening on OSH programmes: effectiveness evaluation of the Wellworks-2 intervention in 15 manufacturing worksites. *Occupational and Environmental Medicine*, **61**, 651–60.

Landsbergis PA, Cahill J, and Schnall PL (1999). The impact of lean production and related new systems of work organization on worker health. *Journal of Occupational Health Psychology*, **4**, 108–30.

Lanoie P and Tavenas S (1996). Costs and benefits of preventing workplace accidents: the case of participatory ergonomics. *Safety Science*, **24**, 181–96.

Laupacis A, Feeny D, Detsky AS, and Tugwell PX (1992). How attractive does a new technology have to be to warrant adoption and utilization? Tentative guidelines for using clinical and economic evaluations. *Canadian Medical Association Journal*, **146**, 473–81.

Lavis JN, Mustard CA, Payne JI, and Farrant MSR (1998). *Employment, working conditions and health: towards a set of population-level indicators.* Toronto: Institute for Work & Health.

Lavis JN, Mustard CA, Payne JI, and Farrant MSR (2001). Work-related population health indicators. *Canadian Journal of Public Health*, **92**, 72–8.

Lawler EE (1975). *Pay, participation, and organizational change. Man and Work in Society.* Van Nostrand Reinhold Co., New York.

Leigh JP and Robbins JA (2004). Occupational disease and workers' compensation: coverage, costs and consequences. *Milbank Quarterly*, **82**, 689–721.

Leigh J, Macaskill P, Corvalan C, Kuosma E, and Mandryk J (1996a). *Global burden of disease and injury due to occupational factors.* Geneva: World Health Organization.

Leigh JP, Markowitz SB, Fahs M, Shin C, and Landrigan PJ (1996b). *Costs of occupational injuries and illnesses.* Cincinnati: NIOSH.

Lerner DJ, Amick III BC, Lee J, Rooney T, Rogers WH, Chang H, Berndt ER (2003). Relationship of employee-reported work limitations to work productivity. *Medical Care*, **41**, 649–59.

Lewis R, Krawiec M, Confer E, Agopsowicz D, and Crandall E (2002). Musculoskeletal disorder worker compensation costs and injuries before and after an office ergonomic program. *International Journal of Industrial Ergonomics*, **29**, 95–9.

Lilienfeld DE and Stolley PD (1994). *Foundations of epidemiology.* Oxford University Press, New York.

Little RJ and Rubin DB (2000). Causal effects in clinical and epidemiological studies via potential outcomes: concepts and analytical approaches. *Annual Review of Public Health*, **21**, 121–45.

Livingstone D (1999). *The education–jobs gap: underemployment or economic democracy.* Garamond Press, Toronto.

Locke (1967). *Two treatises on civil government.* Cambridge University Press, Cambridge.

Loisel P, Lemaire J, Poitras S, *et al.* (2002). Cost–benefit and cost-effectiveness analysis of a disability prevention model for back pain management: a six year follow up study. *Occupational and Environmental Medicine*, **59**, 807–15.

Loomes G (1999). Some lessons from past experiments and some challenges for the future. *Economic Journal*, **109**, 35–45.

Löthgren M and Zethraeus N (2000). Definition, interpretation and calculation of cost-effectiveness acceptability curves. *Health Economics*, **9**, 623–30.

Lowe G (2000). *The quality of work.* Oxford University Press, Toronto.

Luken RA (1985). The emerging role of benefit-cost analysis in the regulatory process at EPA. *Environmental Health Perspectives*, **62**, 373–9.

Macaulay AC, Commanda LE, Freeman WL, Gibson N, McCabe ML, Robbins CM, and Twohig PL (1998). *Responsible research with communities: participatory research in primary care. A policy statement.* North American Primary Care Research Group, Leawood. Available at: www.napcrg.org/exec.html

Machina MJ (1987). Choice under uncertainty: problems solved and unsolved. *Journal of Economic Perspectives*, **1**, 121–54.

Mandelblatt JS, Fryback DG, Weinstein MC, Russell LB, Gold MR, and Hadorn DC (1996). Assessing the effectiveness of health interventions. In MR Gold, LB Russell, JE Siegel, and MC Weinstein (eds) *Cost-effectiveness in health and medicine*. Oxford University Press, New York.

Mann FC and Neff FW (1961). *Managing major change in organizations*. Foundation for Research on Human Behavior, Ann Arbor.

Marmot M and Feeney A (1996). Work and health: implications for individuals and society. In D Blane, E Brunner, and R Wilkinson (eds) *Health and Social Organization*. Routledge, London.

Marsden S, Beardwell C, Shaw J, Wright M, Green N, and McGurry B (2004). *The development of case studies that demonstrate the business benefit of effective management of occupational health and safety*. Health and Safety Executive, London.

Martikainen P, Stansfeld S, Hemingway H, and Marmot M (1999). Determinants of socioeconomic differences in change in physical and mental functioning. *Social Science & Medicine*, **49**, 499–507.

Mason H, Marshall A, Jones-Lee M, and Donaldson C (2006). *Estimating a monetary value of a QALY from existing values of preventing fatalities and serious injuries*. Report to UK NHS National Coordinating Centre for Research Methodology.

Materna BL, Harrington D, Scholz P, *et al.* (2002). Results of an intervention to improve lead safety among painting contractors and their employees. *American Journal of Industrial Medicine*, **41**, 119–30.

Matthews S, Hertzmann C, Ostry A, and Power C (1998). Gender, work roles and psychosocial work characteristics as determinants of health. *Social Science & Medicine*, **46**, 1417–24.

Mauskopf JA, Paul JE, Grant DM, and Stergachis A (1998). The role of cost-consequence analysis in health care decision-making. *Pharmacoeconomics*, **13**, 277–88.

McGregor M and Caro JJ (2006). QALYs: are they helpful to decision makers? *Pharmacoeconomics*, **24**, 947–52.

McGuire A, Henderson J, and Mooney G (1992). *The economics of health care: an introductory text*. Routledge, London.

Mill JS (1965). Principles of political economy with some of their applications to social philosophy, Book II. In JM Robson (ed) *Collected Works of John Stuart Mill, Volume II*. University of Toronto Press, Toronto.

Ministry of Health (1994). *Ontario guidelines for economic analysis of pharmaceutical products*. Ministry of Health, Toronto.

Mishan EJ (1971). Evaluation of life and limb: a theoretical approach. *Journal of Political Economy*, **79**, 687–705.

Mishel LJ, Bernstein J, and Schmitt J (1997). *The state of working America: 1996–1997*. M. E. Sharpe, Armonk.

Mohr DL and Clemmer DI (1989). Evaluation of an occupational injury intervention in the petroleum drilling industry. *Accident Analysis and Prevention*, **21**, 263–71.

Mooney G (1992). *Economics, medicine and health care*. Harvester Wheatsheaf, Hemel Hempstead.

Moore M and Viscusi WK (1988). Workers' compensation: wage effects, benefit inadequacies, and the value of health losses. *Review of Economics and Statistics*, **69**, 249–61.

Morrell S, Taylor R, Quine S, Kerr C, and Western J (1997). A cohort study of unemployment as a cause of psychological disturbance in Australian youth. *Social Science & Medicine*, **38**, 1553–64.

Murray CJL and Lopez AD (1996a). *The global burden of disease*. Harvard University Press, on behalf of the World Health Organization, Cambridge.

Murray CJL and Lopez AD (1996b). The global burden of disease: a comprehensive assessment of mortality and disability from diseases, injuries and risk factors in 1990 and projected to 2020. In *Global burden of disease and injury series, Volume 1*. Harvard University Press, Cambridge.

Mustard CA, Vermeulen M, and Lavis JN (2003). Is position in the occupational hierarchy a determinant of decline in perceived health status? *Social Science & Medicine*, **57**, 2291–303.

Myles J (1988). The expanding middle: some Canadian evidence on the deskilling debate. *Canadian Review of Sociology and Anthropology*, **25**, 335–64.

National Institute for Clinical Excellence (2004). *Guide to the methods of technology appraisal*, London: National Institute for Clinical Excellence.

National Institute for Clinical Excellence (2005). *Assessing evidence and prioritising recommendations in NICE guidance*. London: National Institute for Clinical Excellence.

National Institute for Health & Clinical Excellence (2007). *Social value judgements: principles for the development of NICE guidance, second edition: draft for public consultation*, p. 217. Available at: www.nice.org.uk/aboutnice/howwework/socialvaluejudgements/SVJconsultation.jsp?domedia=1&mid=8B4C7211–19B9-E0B5-D43EC713540B6AB4.

Navarro V (2001). *The political economy of social inequalities: consequences for health and quality of life*. Baywood, New York.

Nerhood H and Rael J (1995). Low tech, low cost approach to office ergonomics. In AC Jr Bittner and PC Champney (eds) *Advances in industrial ergonomics and safety VII*. Taylor and Francis, London, pp. 363–7.

Neumann WP, Forsman M, Kihlberg S, *et al.* (2002). Initiating an ergonomics process—tips, tricks and traps. Commentary from focus groups and case studies. In *Humans in a complex environment: proceedings of the 34th Annual Congress of the Nordic Ergonomics society*. Linkoping University, Division of Industrial Ergonomics, Kolmarden, Sweden.

Ng YK (1983). *Welfare economics: introduction and development of basic concepts*. Macmillan, London.

Nicholson S, Pauly MV, Polsky D, Sharda C, Szrek H, and Berger ML (2006). Measuring the effects of work loss on productivity with team production. *Health Economics*, **15**, 111–23.

Niven KJ (2002). A review of the application of health economics to health and safety in health care. *Health Policy*, **61**, 291–304.

Nozik R (1974). *Anarchy, state and utopia*. Basic Books, New York.

Nurick AJ (1982). Participation in organizational change: a longitudinal field study. *Human Relations*, **35**, 413–29.

Nurminen M and Karjalainen A (2001). Epidemiologic estimate of the proportion of fatalities related to occupational factors in Finland. *Scandinavian Journal of Work, Environment & Health*, **27**, 161–213.

O'Grady J (2000). Joint Health and Safety Committees: finding the balance. In TJ Sullivan (ed) *Injury and the new world of work*. University of British Columbia Press, Vancouver.

O'Hagan A and Stevens JW (2002). Bayesian methods for the design and analysis of cost-effectiveness trials in the evaluation of health care technologies. *Statistical Methods in Medical Research*, **11**, 469–90.

Osterhaus JT, Gutterman DL, and Plachetka JR (1992) Health care resource and lost labour costs of migraine headache in the US. *Pharmacoeconomics*, **2**, 67–76.

Osterman P (1999). *Securing prosperity: the American labor market, how it has been changed, and what to do about it*. Princeton University Press, Princeton.

Ostry A, Marion S, Green LW, *et al.* (2000). Downsizing and industrial restructuring in related to changes in psychosocial conditions of work in British Columbia sawmills. *Scandinavian Journal of Work, Environment & Health*, **26**, 273–8.

Oxenburgh M, Marlow P and Oxenburgh A (2004). *Increasing productivity and profit through health and safety: the financial returns from a safe working environment*, (2nd edn). CRC Press, Boca Raton.

Palley TI (1998). *Plenty of nothing*. Princeton University Press, Princeton.

Paoli P and Merllie D (2001). *Third European Survey on working conditions*. European Foundation for the Improvement of Living and Working Conditions. Dublin, Report No. EF/01/21.

Parkin D and Devlin N (2006). Is there a case for using visual analogue scale valuations in Cost Utility Analysis? *Health Economics*, **15**, 653–64.

Pauly MV (1995). Valuing health care benefits in money terms. In FA Sloan (ed) *Valuing health care. Costs, benefits and effectiveness of pharmaceuticals and other medical technologies*. Cambridge University Press, Cambridge, pp. 99–124.

Pauly MV, Nicholson S, Xu J, *et al.* (2002). A general model of the impact of absenteeism on employees. *Health Economics*, **11**, 221–31.

Petty W (1899). Verbum Sapienti. In CH Hall (ed) *The economic writings of Sir William Petty*. Routledge/Thoemmes, London.

Plant R (1991). *Modern political thought*. Basil Blackwell, Oxford.

Polanyi MF and Cole DC (2003). Stakeholder engagement in the control of repetitive strain injury. In Sullivan T and Frank J (eds) *Preventing and managing disabling injury at work*. Taylor & Francis, New York, pp. 125–141.

Pollin R and Luce S (1998). *The living wage: building a fair economy*. New Press, New York.

Power C and Hertzman C (1997). Social and biological pathways linking early life and adult disease. *British Medical Bulletin*, **53**, 210–21.

Pritchard C and Sculpher M (2000). *Productivity costs: principles and practice in economic evaluation*. Office of Health Economics, London.

Quinlan M (1998). Labour market restructuring in industrialised societies: an overview. *Economic and Labour Relations Review*, **9**, 1–30.

Quinlan M, Mayhew C, and Bohle P (2001). The global expansion of precarious employment, work disorganization, and consequences for occupational health: a review of recent research. *International Journal of Health Services*, **31**, 335–414.

Rawlins MD and Culyer AJ (2004). National Institute for Clinical Excellence and its value judgments. *British Medical Journal*, **329**, 224–7.

Rawls J (1971). *A theory of justice*. Harvard University Press, Cambridge.

Rees J (1988). Self regulation: an effective alternative to direct regulation by OSHA? *Policy Studies Journal*, **16**, 602–14.

Reich R (1996). *The work of nations*. Vintage Books, New York.

Rempel DM, Krause N, Goldberg R, Benner D, Hudes M, Goldner GU (2006). A randomised controlled trail evaluating the effects of two workstation interventions on upper body pain and incident musculoskeletal disorders among computer operators. *Occupational and Environmental Medicine*, **63**, 300–6.

Richardson D (2002). Ergonomics and retention. *Caring*, **21**, 6–9.

Rifkin J (1996). *The end of work: the decline of the global labor force and the dawn of the post-market era*. Putnam, New York.

Rivilis I, Van Eerd D, Cullen K, *et al.* (2008). Effectiveness of participatory ergonomic interventions o health outcomes: a systematic review. *Applied Ergonomics*, **39**, 342–58.

Robson LS, Cole DC, Shannon HS, and the Healthy Workplace Group (2005). *Healthy workplace performance measurement*. Institute for Work & Health, Toronto, Working Paper # 256.

Rosen S (1986). Theory of equalizing differences. In O Ashenfelter and R Layard (eds) *Handbook of labor economics, V1*, pp. 641–92. North Holland, New York.

Rosenbaum PR (1995). *Observational studies*. Springer-Verlag, New York.

Rosenbaum PR and Rubin DB (1983). The central role of the propensity score in observational studies for causal effects. *Biometrica*, **70**, 41–55.

Rothman KJ and Greenland S (1998). *Modern epidemiology*. Lippincott-Raven, Philadelphia.

Rubin DB (1991). Practical implications of modes of statistical inference for causal effects and the critical role of the assignment mechanism. *Biometrics*, **47**, 1213–34.

Schulte PA (2005). Characterizing the burden of occupational injury and disease. *Journal of Occupational and Environmental Medicine*, **47**, 607–22.

Sculpher M and Drummond M (2006). Analysis sans frontières: can we ever make economic evaluations generalisable across jurisdictions? *Pharmacoeconomics*, **24**, 1087–99.

Sculpher M, Claxton K, and Akehurst R (2005). It's just evaluation for decision making: recent developments in, and challenges for, cost-effectiveness research. In PC Smith, L Ginnelly, and M Sculpher (eds) *Health policy and economics. Opportunities and challenges*. Open University Press, Maidenhead, pp. 8–41.

Sen A (1980). *Commodities and capabilities*. Oxford University Press, Oxford.

Sen A (1993). Capability and well-being. In M Nussbaum and A Sen (eds) *The quality of life*. Clarendon Press, Oxford, pp. 30–53.

Shadish WR, Cook TD, and Campbell DT (2002). *Experimental and quasi-experimental designs for generalized causal inference*. Houghton Mifflin, Boston.

Shannon HS and Lowe GS (2002). How many injured workers do not file claims for workers' compensation benefits? *American Journal of Industrial Medicine*, **42**, 467–73.

Shannon HS, Robson LS, and Guastello SJ (1999). Methodological criteria for evaluation occupational safety intervention research. *Safety Science*, **31**, 161–79.

Shikiar R, Halpern M, Rentz A, and Khan Z (2004). Development of the Health and Work Questionnaire (HWQ): an instrument for assessing workplace productivity in relation to worker health. *Work*, **22**, 219–29.

Shogren JF and Stamland T (2002). Skill and the value of life. *Journal of Political Economy*, **110**, 1168–73.

Shumway M (2003). Preference weights for cost-outcome analyses of schizophrenia treat-ments: comparison of four stakeholder groups. *Schizophrenia Bulletin*, **29**, 257–66.

Siegrist J and Marmot M (2004). Health inequalities and the psychosocial environment—two scientific challenges. *Social Science & Medicine*, **58**, 1463–73.

Simon GE, Katon WJ, Von Korff M, *et al.* (2001). Cost-effectiveness of a collaborative care program for primary care patients with persistent depression. *American Journal of Psychiatry*, **158**, 1638–44.

Smallman C and John G (2001). British directors' perspectives on the impact of health and safety on corporate performance. *Safety Science*, **38**, 227–39.

Smulders PGW, Kompier MAJ, and Paoli P (1996). The work environment in the twelve EU-countries: differences and similarities. *Human Relations*, **49**, 1291–313.

Solow RM (1990). *The labor market as a social institution.* Basil Blackwell, Cambridge.

Sorlie PD and Rogot E (1990). Mortality by employment status in the National Longitudinal Mortality Study. *American Journal of Epidemiology*, **132**, 983–92.

Spiegelhalter DJ, Abrams KR, and Myles JP (2004). *Bayesian approaches to clinical trials and health-care evaluation.* John Wiley & Sons Ltd., West Sussex.

Steenland L, Burnett C, Lalich N, Ward E, and Hurrell J (2003). Dying for work: the magnitude of US mortality from selected causes of death associated with occupation. *American Journal of Industrial Medicine*, **43**, 461–82.

Stewart WF, Ricci JA, Chee E, Morganstein D, and Lipton R (2003). Lost productive time and cost due to common pain conditions in the US workforce. *Journal of the American Medical Association*, **290**, 2443–54.

Stinnett AA and Paltiel AD (1996). Mathematical programming for the efficient allocation of health care resources. *Journal of Health Economics*, **15**, 641–53.

Sugden R and Williams A (1978). *The principles of practical cost–benefit analysis.* Oxford University Press, Oxford.

Tadano P (1990). A safety/prevention program for VDT operators: one company's approach. *Journal of Hand Therapy*, **3**, 64–71.

Tarn TY and Smith MD (2005). Pharmacoeconomic guidelines around the world. *ISPOR Connections*, **10**, 5.

Theorell T (1999). How to deal with stress in organizations? A health perspective on theory and practice. *Scandinavian Journal of Work, Environment & Health*, **25**, 616–24.

Thompson DA (1990). Effect of exercise breaks on musculoskeletal strain among data-entry operators: a case study. In M Dainoff (ed) *Promoting health and productivity in the com-puterized office: models of successful ergonomic interventions.* Taylor & Francis, London.

Tompa E, Dolinschi R, and de Oliveira C (2006). Practice and potential of economic evaluation of workplace-based interventions for occupational health and safety. *Journal of Occupational Rehabilitation*, **16**, 375–400.

Tompa E, Dolinschi R, de Oliveira C, and Irvin E (2007a). *A systematic review of OHS interventions with economic evaluations.* Toronto: Institute for Work & Health.

Tompa E, Dolinschi R, de Oliveira C, and Irvin E (2007b). *Final report on a systematic review of OHS interventions with economic evaluations.* Toronto: Institute for Work & Health.

Tompa E, Scott-Marshall H, Dolinschi R, Trevithick S, and Bhattacharyya S (2007c). Precarious employment experiences and their health consequences: towards a theoretical framework. *Work: a Journal of Prevention, Assessment and Rehabilitation*, **28**, 209–24.

Viscusi WK (1992). *Fatal tradeoffs: public and private responsibilities for risk*. Oxford University Press, New York.

Viscusi WK (1993). The value of risks to life and health. *Journal of Economic Literature*, **31**, 1912–46.

Viscusi WK and Aldy J (2003). The value of a statistical life: a critical review of market estimates throughout the world. *Journal of Risk and Uncertainty*, **27**, 5–76.

Viscusi WK and Aldy JE (2005). *The value of a statistical life: a critical review of market estimates throughout the world*. National Bureau of Economic Research, Inc., Cambridge, Working Paper # 9487.

Wadsworth MEJ, Montgomery SM, and Bartley MJ (1999). The persisting effect of unemployment on health and social well-being in men early in working life. *Social Science & Medicine*, **48**, 1491–9.

Wagstaff A and van Doorslaer E (2000). Equity in health care finance and delivery. In AJ Culyer and JP Newhouse (eds) *Handbook of health economics*. Elsevier, Amsterdam, pp. 1803–62.

Weil D (2001). Valuing the economic consequences of work injury and illness: a comparison of methods and findings. *American Journal of Industrial Medicine*, **40**, 418–37.

Weinstein M and Zeckhauser R (1973). Critical ratios and efficient allocation. *Journal of Public Economics*, **2**, 147–58.

Weinstein MC, Siegel JE, Garber AM, Lipscomb J, Luce BR, Manning Jr. WG and Torrance GW (1997). Productivity costs, time costs and health-related quality of life: a response to the Erasmus group. *Health Economics*, **6**, 505–10.

Williams A (1997). The rationing debate: rationing health care by age: the case for. *British Medical Journal*, **314**, 820.

Williams A and Cookson R (2000). Equity in health. In AJ Culyer and JP Newhouse (eds) *Handbook of health economics*. Elsevier, Amsterdam, pp. 1863–1910.

Woodward C, Shannon H, Cunningham C, *et al.* (1999). The impact of re-engineering and other cost reduction strategies on the staff of a large teaching hospital. *Medical Care*, **37**, 556–69.

Workplace Safety and Insurance Board and Canadian Manufacturers and Exporters (2002). *Business results through health & safety*. Workplace Safety & Insurance Board, Toronto.

Yassi A, Khokhar J, Tate R, Cooper J, Snow C, and Vallentyne S (1995a). The epidemiology of back injuries in nurses at a large Canadian tertiary care hospital: implications for prevention. *Occupational Medicine*, **45**, 215–20.

Yassi A, Tate R, Cooper JE, Snow C, Vallentyne S, and Khokhar JB (1995b). Early intervention for back-injured nurses at a large Canadian tertiary care hospital: an evaluation of the effectiveness and cost benefits of a two-year pilot project. *Occupational Medicine*, **45**, 209–14.

Zaza S, Wright-De Aguero LK, Briss PA, *et al.* (2000). Data collection instrument and procedure for systematic reviews in the Guide to Community Preventive Services. Task Force on Community Preventive Services. *American Journal of Preventive Medicine*, **18(1S)**, 44–74.

Zwerling C, Daltroy LH, Fine LJ, Johnston JJ, Melius J, and Silverstein BA (1997). Design and conduct of occupational injury intervention studies: a review of evaluation strategies. *American Journal of Industrial Medicine*, **32**, 164–79.

Author Index

Subject Index

Please note bold entries are page numbers for terms that have been defined in the glossary